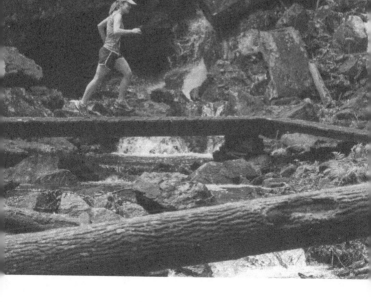

TRAIL
RUNNING
ERN
NT

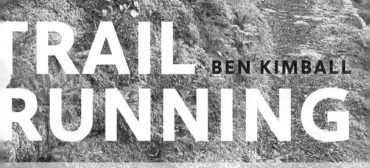

TRAIL
RUNNING

BEN KIMBALL

SOUTHERN
VERMONT

Trail Running Southern Vermont has been supported by the Regional
Books Fund, established by donors in 2019 to support the University
of Massachusetts Press's Bright Leaf imprint.

Bright Leaf, an imprint of the University of Massachusetts Press, publishes
accessible and entertaining books about New England. Highlighting the
history, culture, diversity, and environment of the region, Bright Leaf offers
readers the tools and inspiration to explore its landmarks and traditions,
famous personalities, and distinctive flora and fauna.

ISBN 978-1-62534-789-3 (paper)

Designed by Deste Roosa
Set in Quadraat
Printed and bound by Books International, Inc.

Cover design by Deste Roosa
Cover photo by David S. Jenne, Trail runner at Pine Hill Park in Rutland, Vermont, 2018.
Courtesy of the photographer | photography.davidjenne.com.

Library of Congress Cataloging-in-Publication Data

Names: Kimball, Ben, author.
Title: Trail running Southern Vermont / Ben Kimball.
Description: Amherst : Bright Leaf, An imprint of University of
   Massachusetts Press, 2024. | Identifiers: LCCN 2023046500 (print) | LCCN
2023046501 (ebook) | ISBN
   9781625347893 (paperback) | ISBN 9781685750640 (ebook) | ISBN
9781685750657 (ebook)
Subjects: LCSH: Mountain running—Vermont—Guidebooks. |
   Trails—Vermont—Guidebooks. | Vermont—Guidebooks.
Classification: LCC GV1061.22.V4 K56 2024 (print) | LCC GV1061.22.V4
   (ebook) | DDC 796.5109743—dc23/eng/20231103
LC record available at https://lccn.loc.gov/2023046500
LC ebook record available at https://lccn.loc.gov/2023046501

British Library Cataloguing-in-Publication Data
A catalog record for this book is available from the British Library.

Portions of the introduction were previously published in Trail Running Eastern
Massachusetts (Amherst: University of Massachusetts Press, 2022). Copyright © 2022
University of Massachusetts Press.

Figure 1. Running below The Falls at Ascutney Trails.
Figure 2. The West Ridge Trail near Bennington.
Figure 3. Running the Last Mile path at Ascutney Trails.

All photos and maps by Ben Kimball.

Contents

Figures

Acknowledgments

This guide was created with the support and assistance of countless friends in the regional running community. My awesome partner, Jennifer Garrett, once again helped with everything, including research, logistics, and manuscript editing, not to mention endless encouragement. Others who provided invaluable advice, insight, or company include Donald Campbell, Alison Clarkson, Stephen Engle, Josh Fields, Stephan Fowlkes, Greg Hanscom, Roger Haydock, Jack Jessup, Alex Jospe, Michael Paulsen, Tom and Laure Van den Broeck Raffensperger, Fred Ross, Amy Rusiecki, Jason Sarouhan, Alex Shaffer, Garth Shaneyfelt, and Deb Shearer. Many organizations and resources proved useful for researching trails, including the Vermont Department of Forests, Parks and Recreation (FPR), various land trusts and conservation groups, and several online mapping sites. All profiled routes were visited and mapped in person, however, and any errors in them are entirely my own. Most of the base-map layers were obtained from Vermont Center for Geographic Information and various municipalities. Thanks also to the terrific production staff at UMass Press; they ensured every stage of this project ran very smoothly. Finally, special thanks to the local conservation organizations, land trusts, recreation departments, hiking clubs, mountain bike clubs, friends groups, and volunteers who help build and maintain the wonderful trails of southern Vermont.

SITE LOCATIONS

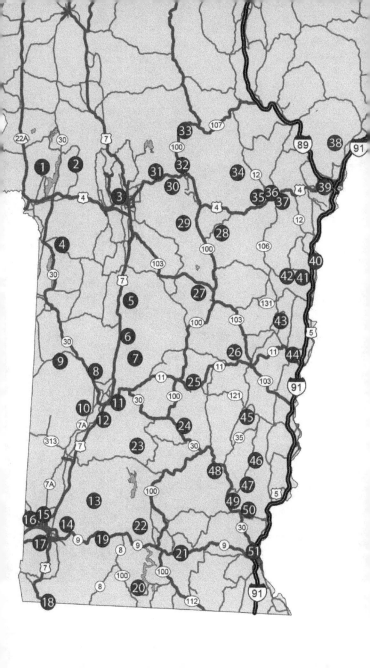

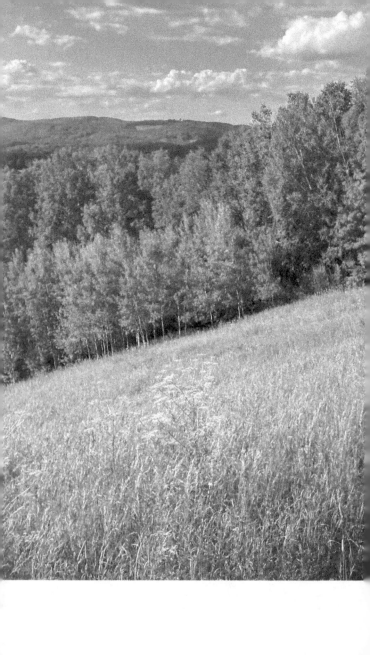

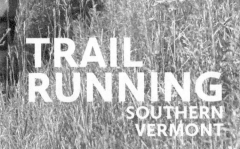

TRAIL
RUNNING
SOUTHERN
VERMONT

Introduction

Whether swiftly gliding through the woods, leaping over fallen logs, or soaring along scenic mountain ridges, trail runners always seem to be enjoying themselves. This is hardly surprising, since trail running combines the best aspects of many healthy and enjoyable activities. Among other things, it provides opportunities for achieving good fitness workouts, spending time outdoors exploring new terrain, and connecting to the natural landscape in a direct and personal way. The appeal of trail racing has become apparent to the broader running community, and the sport remains extremely popular.

Trail running is a particularly tactile experience, constantly forcing you to be mindful and aware of the world around you. Since it frequently requires the body to balance and stabilize itself, it strengthens different sets of muscles than running on pavement and generally results in less impact on the legs.

No special gear is needed, though certain specially designed items can greatly increase enjoyment, performance, and safety. Trail-running shoes often feature aggressive soles that improve grip and comfort in various conditions such as mud, grass, and loose rocks; handheld water bottles or hydration packs/vests can be very helpful on longer runs, or even shorter runs in warm weather; and extra traction is frequently useful in winter.

Hiking is often a natural part of trail running for most people, especially on steep slopes where hiking may even be more efficient. By integrating running with hiking on trails, you can cover more miles in less time, but this also means you may move more quickly past sights. It's a balancing act, but with experience running can be just as rewarding an outdoor experience. You also feel the ground differently while trail running—flowing over it rather than just stepping on it—and you make crucial, split-second decisions about where to place your feet with each stride.

SOUTHERN VERMONT TRAIL SITES The rural and sometimes wild landscape of the Southern Vermont region offers a true bounty of great trail-running opportunities, from out-and-back (or point-to-point) runs on popular long-distance routes, such as the Long Trail and the Appalachian Trail, to little-known loops hidden away in the woods. Even near the more populated areas, you can find plenty of places where runners can roam for miles.

The intent of this guide is to present a diverse selection of enjoyable runs in the region. It features many sites for experienced runners seeking less traveled but still interesting and fun trails away from the beaten path, and it aims to be inclusive, with a number of easily accessible sites for anyone looking for first-step exposure to trail running. However, it generally avoids short paths at smaller sites, loops shorter than two or three miles, and paved or partly paved pathways. Naturally, there are hundreds more sites where you can find good local trail-running options if you do multiple loops on shorter trails or link smaller sites together. Local schools often have great cross-country trail networks nearby, too.

Geographically, the book covers the area from a bit north of Rte. 4 south to the Massachusetts state line. Elevations range from lows in the Connecticut River Valley to over 4,000 feet at Killington Peak. The trails profiled also represent a range of difficulty levels and terrain types. Other factors considered in final site selection included legal public access, current condition, and adequate parking.

Broadly speaking, the sites are spread relatively evenly throughout the region, with a few notable exceptions. The Woodstock, Manchester, and Bennington areas are particularly rich in good, publicly accessible trail running sites. Conversely, some of the wilder parts of the Green Mountain National Forest are intentionally trail-free, and a few trail systems specifically prohibit running. Also of note: the course routes for several of the area's most popular ultramarathon events, including Vermont 100 and Vermont 50, run on private land and are not open to the public except on race day.

There are options here for everyone. However, these are still only a sampling; there are *many* other trails out there to explore—including some more great ones just waiting for you to discover them. Make sure to check each site's "Nearby" section for a few ideas.

LONG-DISTANCE TRAILS AND RAIL TRAILS While this book specifically profiles fifty-one of the best trail-running sites in southern Vermont, other good options can be found along almost any portion of the region's most prominent long-distance routes, like the Long Trail (272 miles) and the Appalachian Trail (150 miles in VT). For example, the sections north and south of Clarendon Gorge and White Rocks, while occasionally steep and rugged, are fun to explore. Official websites offer detailed maps and information.

Likewise, the region's unpaved rail-trail corridors, which can be accessed from multiple locations, offer easy running routes that are good for beginner trail runners or anyone looking for gentle out-and-back runs on flat to rolling dirt surfaces. These include the Delaware and Hudson (D&H) Rail Trail in Castleton/Poultney and West Pawlett/Rupert; the northern section of the Hoot, Toot & Whistle Rail Trail in Wilmington/Readsboro; the Historic Marble Rail Trail in Manchester; and the lower portion of the West River Trail in Brattleboro/Dummerston, among others. Some portions of the long-distance Catamount Trail (a cross-country ski trail) are also runnable in summer, though overall it is not specifically maintained for summer use and parts may be impassable.

BEGINNER-FRIENDLY TRAILS This book includes a number of profiled sites with suggested routes that are well-suited for beginners or those seeking easier runs. Examples include Mile-Around Woods, Lake Paran, Lowell Lake, and Woodford State Park, as well as almost any part of the West River Trail and some of the easier loops at Pine Hill Park, Slate Valley Trails, Sherburne Trails, and Paradise Park. Additionally, a few other sites that would make great introductory places for first-timers to try out trail running would be the Bill Ballard Trail in Norwich, the mile-long trail around Hapgood Pond in Peru, and Mount Peg or The Pogue in Woodstock.

CONSERVATION Trail running's continued rise in popularity brings increased environmental impact on the beautiful pathways and landscapes we all love to escape to. By promoting and practicing low-impact mindsets and suggesting best practices for treading lightly, we can try to preserve these treasured resources for generations to come.

Avoid running on trails when they're most vulnerable, particularly in spring. As the snow melts from a long New England winter, everyone wants to get out and hit the trails; unfortunately, this is when the impact from running can do the most damage. Ground saturated with snowmelt is soft and easily eroded, and formerly pleasant paths can quickly become ruts of exposed roots and rocks. Staying off the trails during the wettest weeks will help ensure that they remain in top shape for the rest of the year.

Vermont's famous "Mud Season" generally spans the lengthy period in the spring between snowmelt and Memorial Day. During this time, many trails may be officially closed by land managers; please respect any signage or postings you see. Many trail networks are built and maintained by volunteer groups that are run by donation; damage done during wet periods can be costly to repair.

Beyond avoiding the most vulnerable times of year, it's also preferable to stick to the middle of existing trails—even if that means encountering a mud puddle or two—rather than going off to the side, which widens trails and unnecessarily hastens erosion. Finally, *never* cut off a switchback in the trail; they're there specifically to lessen the grade and prevent erosion.

Dispersing is another way to reduce impact. Instead of always visiting a favorite popular trail, consider going to such places only on weekdays when crowds are smaller and using your weekends to explore more remote, less visited sites. Not only will you decrease use

Perhaps most importantly, you can get involved with conservation organizations that are committed to preserving and maintaining stewardship over natural areas and publicly accessible lands with trails. There are many excellent local "friends" groups, clubs, and associations in southern Vermont that you can support with financial pledges or service hours; a lot of them host volunteer maintenance workdays where you can help out and keep the trails in top condition.

ETIQUETTE Observing several basic rules of behavior will go a long way toward fostering goodwill with landowners and land managers and helping to ensure continued public access to a wide variety of trails. The more we present a positive image of runners as respectful and responsible users of trails, the better an experience everyone will have and the more welcome we'll be in the future.

Encounters with other users are virtually guaranteed, even at the remotest of sites. Always be courteous of hikers, bikers, equestrian riders, and other runners, making way whenever possible. Also, never underestimate the powerful good vibes that can be generated by a simple "hello" or friendly nod to a fellow trail user. If you encounter a motorized off-road vehicle such as an all-terrain vehicle or motorbike, you as a pedestrian have the right-of-way—technically. But demonstrate kindness and step aside for them anyway, especially on any trails specifically designated for their use; you will likely hear them long before they see you anyway.

Mountain bikes are allowed at most sites unless otherwise noted, though some trails are posted as off-limits. Likewise, dogs are allowed at many sites; exceptions are indicated in the text. If you run with a dog, it should always be leashed (except in designated areas) or kept under proper control, especially as you approach other dogs and trail users.

Finally, bear in mind that while many trail networks (such as those in state parks and forests) were designed for a variety of recreational uses, others specifically encourage quiet and passive uses. For example, running is specifically prohibited on trails at most properties managed by The Nature Conservancy in Vermont; for that reason, none are included here. At properties where running is allowed but the primary purpose is conservation, please take extra care to not disturb wildlife or native vegetation, or other visitors who are there specifically to enjoy those things.

SAFETY While there are a number of factors to consider when planning a trail run, none is more important than hydration: you simply have to have enough water. There are dozens of handheld water bottles and hydration packs on the market in which you can carry water, sports drinks, whatever. Experiment with what works best for you; just make sure you drink. One note of caution: never drink untreated water from an untested source.

Insects are probably the most common animals you'll encounter. Extra clothing or bug repellent deters mosquitoes and blackflies, which can be maddening in large numbers, especially in the days following summer rainstorms. Tick checks are a must after any run through shrubby or grassy areas. Wasps, hornets, and yellowjackets may also be encountered. Your best defense against them is to be on the lookout for nests, but should you accidentally stir some up or find yourself getting stung, just do what comes naturally: run away as fast as you can.

Encounters with large mammals are rare, but you may see deer, moose, or black bears. A black bear will typically run away should you happen upon one, but if it doesn't, back away and leave it be if possible or make noise and try to look big if it appears threatening. In more remote areas, you might see a moose. Moose rarely charge, but it's best to stay out of their way and observe from a distance, just in case. Note that seasonal hunting is permitted on many of the properties profiled in this book. For up-to-date hunting-season information, check with the Vermont Fish & Wildlife Department, and if you'll be running during an open season, wear bright orange clothing.

Naturally, trail runners must take care to avoid falls and physical injuries such as sprained ankles while out in the woods. Potential hazards to watch out for include wet rocks or ledges, wet or slippery leaves, wet wooden boardwalks or bridges, and slopes covered in loose gravel. Practicing mindfulness and slowing your pace appropriately while making your way along a rough section of trail are necessary to ensure safe foot placement as you travel over the constantly changing terrain.

Trail runners should also be aware of poison ivy; make sure you know what it looks like and where it tends to grow. Poison ivy often thrives in disturbed areas and can be particularly dense right along the edges of roads, trails, and rivers, especially at lower elevations. Usually you can step over or pick your way through a patch along a trail, but a slight detour may be called for on occasion.

Always leave early enough in the day to make it back to the trailhead by nightfall unless you plan to run with a headlamp. Also, check the weather forecast before heading out, particularly for remote sites or if taking trails that ascend to higher elevations. Prepare for the worst conditions possible and be willing to change your plans based on changes in the weather—even if it means cutting your run short. When it's wet and chilly out, be watchful for any early warning signs of hypothermia, such as cold feet and hands, pale skin, shivering, fatigue, or slurred speech. Hypothermia can be especially dangerous in temperatures just above freezing. It's good practice to carry a lightweight jacket, extra water, snacks, gloves, and a headlamp with you on longer trail runs, just in case. Lastly, always tell someone your intended route and an estimated return time, if possible. Cell service is patchy in this region and should not be counted on.

Unfortunately, other humans can sometimes be a danger on the trails; the threat is rare, but real. Women in particular have been the target of harassment and violence, and many choose to run with friends, carry personal defense items, or learn about self-defense strategies.

Nature, and by extension the trails we run, should be a refuge for all. As in many spaces in American society, people of color, LGBTQ folks, and people with disabilities have at times been made to feel uncomfortable or unwelcome at races or in public parks. We all bear responsibility to create a welcoming and safe environment for everyone. The trails are for all.

TRAIL ACCESS   All the trails profiled in this guide are open to the public. Most are on public land, but occasional portions cross privately-owned parcels and a few sites are entirely on private land open to the public with permission. When following publicly accessible trails that cross private property, always respect the rights and desires of the landowners. Obey all posted notices, especially any "No Trespassing" signs, and never intentionally move or damage structures such as fences or gates. Only currently open trails were included at the time of this guide's writing, but users should be aware that trail closures or re-routings (or both) are possible at any time.

Each site described sits on land which has served as places of meeting and exchange among Indigenous peoples since long before Western settlement of North America. As I run through these beautiful forests and along their rushing rivers today, I challenge myself to remember the connection the Abenaki people have to this region, acknowledge the hardships they've endured and continue to experience, and be thankful for the opportunity to enjoy all the pleasures the natural landscape has to offer us.

REPEATED NAMES   Several geographic place names get repeated multiple times in southern Vermont. Green Mountain, for starters. The Green Mountains run north–south through the center of the state, and the Green Mountain National Forest covers much (but not all) of that mountain chain. There are also several individual peaks named Green Mountain, as well as several *former* Green Mountain summits now renamed something else. In addition, several organizations use the name, including the Green Mountain Club (GMC), Green Mountain Conservancy (also GMC), and Green Mountain Trails (GMT). It's easy to mix them up. Another name that shows up multiple times is Bald Mountain; there are two described as profiled sites in this book (in Bennington and Townshend) as well as several others that appear as Nearby sites, like the one near Bellows Falls and the one in Mendon. The landscape was largely denuded of forest about a century ago and many hilltops were either barren or covered in pasture, so the names actually make plenty of sense even though none of the summits remain bald today. Other duplicate names to be aware of include Mount Tom, White Rocks, Bare Mountain, Bear Mountain, Haystack, Spruce Peak, and Pinnacle, among others. Curiously this is not an issue with The Darning Needle, a 2,883-foot peak in Chittenden, or Bloodsucker Pond in Springfield.

HOW TO USE THIS BOOK Each trail-running route in this book has a chapter dedicated to it, as numbered on the locator map. Each site profile begins with quick-reference data for easily determining if it's suitable for your running ambitions on a given day, including:

Distance: total mileage of the suggested route

Town: municipality(s) the site is in

Difficulty Rating: subjective categories of easy, moderate, and challenging (or combinations)

Trail Style: shape of the route on a map, including loop, lollipop (a loop with a "stick" portion), out-and-back, and figure-8

Trail Type: width and character of the trail itself; includes singletrack, doubletrack, and dirt road

Total Ascent: cumulative elevation gain (best estimation) of the entire primary suggested route

This basic data is followed by a general description of that profile's route, highlighting some of the standout features you'll encounter there. Next comes directions to the trailhead from the nearest town or highway and GPS search suggestions.

The bulk of each chapter is given over to detailed, sometimes turn-by-turn trail descriptions of the route itself that—along with a judicious use of the maps contained in this book—should get you from start to finish without making a wrong turn or becoming mystifyingly lost in the wilderness. These sections often include optional extensions for lengthening a given run or—alternatively—trims for shortening if you don't want to tackle the entire trail that day.

Finally, each site profile spotlights other *nearby* sites that are good for trail running (there's a lot more than fifty-one!).

TERMINOLOGY   Trail running uses some descriptive lingo that general readers (and some runners) may not be familiar with. The following frequently used terms appear throughout the profiles:

4-way intersection: a crossing of two trails
Bootleg trail: an unofficial trail or faint "trace" path
Braid: when a trail splits then later comes back together
Doubletrack: a trail wide enough for two people side-by-side
Fork: like a Y-junction, only with two of the trails tighter together
Lollipop loop: loop route that starts/ends with an out-and-back stem
Runnable: a highly subjective term indicating "not too steep or rough"
Saddle: low point or notch between two summits
Singletrack: a trail wide enough for one person
Switchback: a tight S or Z where the trail changes direction on an ascent or descent
Technical: a trail with more rocks and roots than dirt, often with steep pitches
T-junction: when one trail ends at another; perpendicular to it
Woods/logging/Class IV road: similar to doubletrack, but slightly wider
Y-junction: a 3-way intersection, often with equal angles

DISTANCE 10.2 Miles   **TOWNS** Castleton, Fair Haven, Hubbardton, and Benson
DIFFICULTY RATING Moderate   **TRAIL STYLE** Out-and-Back
TRAIL TYPE Singletrack   **TOTAL ASCENT** 1,090 Feet

The Glen Lake Trail connects Bomoseen State Park with adjacent Half Moon Pond State Park to the north. Blazed with blue markers, it winds through a mix of forest types and visits undeveloped pond shores, remote wetlands, and scenic vistas along the way. This suggested route follows the trail one way north; there is no official trailhead parking at the northern end but it is possible to park along the roadside there. The broader terrain in the region consists of rolling, north–south ridges of the northern Taconic Mountains, with numerous rocky wetlands dotting the landscape, along with occasional old slate quarries and their associated rocky rubble piles. A short trail near the boat launch parking lot explores some of the area's local slate mining history.

DIRECTIONS   From Rte. 4, Exit 3 in Fair Haven, take Scotch Hill Road north for 4 miles. Bear left onto Moscow Road and go 0.1 mile north to the dirt roadside parking lot for Bomoseen State Park's Glen Lake Access Area on the right/east side of the road.

GPS: "74 Moscow Road, Fair Haven, Vermont"

TRAIL   From the sign at the boat access across from the parking area, follow the path west past a line of boulders to a rocky ledge on the shore of Glen Lake. At a sign saying "Glen Lake Trail 4.5 mi." head north on the trail, which rises and falls under cedars, maples, and hemlocks along the eastern shore of the lake. In 0.5 miles, turn left on the unpaved Said Road and go 0.15 miles north. Turn left back onto the trail and go 0.15 miles south back to the edge of the lake. Bear right and go 0.15 miles west to a spur path leading left to

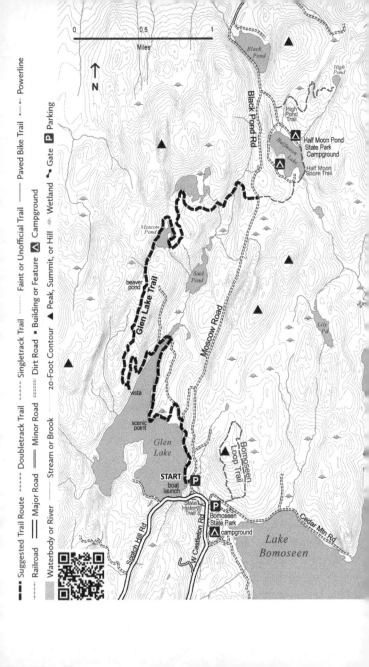

Suggested Trail Route ·••· Doubletrack Trail ----- Singletrack Trail ······ Faint or Unofficial Trail —— Paved Bike Trail •—• Powerline

+++ Railroad ══ Major Road ══ Minor Road ::::::: Dirt Road ——— 20-Foot Contour ▲ Peak, Summit, or Hill ● Building or Feature ▲ Campground ● Gate P Parking

〰 Waterbody or River ——— Stream or Brook 〜 Wetland

0   0.5   1
Miles

↑ N

Black Pond

High Pond

Black Pond Rd

High Pond Trail

▲

Half Moon Pond State Park Campground

Halfmoon Lake

Half Moon Shore Trail

▲

Moscow Pond

Moscow Road

Saüd Pond

▲

Lily Pd

beaver pond

Glen Lake Trail

▲

vista

scenic point

Glen Lake

▲

Bomoseen Loop Trail

START

boat launch

P

Slate History Trail

P

Bomoseen State Park campground

▲

Cedar Mtn Rd

Scotch Hill Rd

W Castleton Rd

Lake Bomoseen

a rocky point. Crossing occasional boardwalks and tackling a few steep pitches, go 0.6 miles north along the east shore of the lake.

Turn left on the dirt road and cross the partially vegetated causeway to the west side of the lake, then bear left and head south along the shore. In 0.15 miles, the trail curves right and begins climbing the hillside. In 0.5 miles it arrives at a junction where a spur path leads a few hundred feet left over to a wide vista at a clearing overlooking Glen Lake and northern hills of the Taconics.

From the junction, follow Glen Lake Trail north away from the water, rising gradually through the woods for about a mile and tracing the edge of a recently harvested area. The trail passes a small, unnamed pond on the left on a hemlock-covered rocky ledge, then arrives at the western side of Moscow Pond. This area can get somewhat flooded in wet years. Go north for about 0.25 miles along the west side of the pond. At the northern end of the pond, the trail swings right and heads south for 0.25 miles along a bluff above the pond to an overlook at the top of a ledge east of the pond; this would make a great spot for a snack.

After the Moscow Pond vista, curve left and go 0.5 miles north to a beaverized wetland. The trail then swings sharply right away from the wetland and heads south. From the wetland, follow the trail 0.9 miles east to Black Pond Road. Along the way the trail crosses several woodland streams and drops steeply to a ravine. It follows the edge of the ravine briefly, crosses it, and then climbs back up out on the other side.

At Black Pond Road, either return the way you came or make a shorter loop by going south along the dirt road. It is 2 miles down to the Glen Lake Access parking area; the road loop option totals 7.1 miles.

Optional Extension From the Moscow Road crossing, extra miles may be added by following Glen Lake Trail 0.4 miles east across a field and then down through the woods to the southern shore of

Half Moon Pond. Take a right at a junction and follow Half Moon Shore Trail 0.4 miles north along the east side of the pond to the campground. Then follow the campground road 0.25 miles north up to the trailhead for High Pond Trail on the right. It is 0.9 miles east from there up to the west edge of scenic High Pond. Total one-way trail length from Glen Lake to High Pond is 7 miles.

NEARBY From the Bomoseen State Park main entrance, the 1.6-mile **Bomoseen Loop Trail** climbs steeply up a hill and loops back to form a lollipop loop. Several miles to the southeast, a short, easy loop can be made on the **Spartan Trail** from a trailhead near the disc-golf course on the west side of Castleton University; from there, the flat **D&H Rail Trail** leads south to Poultney. Note that running is not allowed on the hiking trails of nearby TNC preserves in Benson and West Haven.

DISTANCE 4.2 Miles   **TOWN** Castleton

DIFFICULTY RATING Moderate   **TRAIL STYLE** Figure-8 Loop

TRAIL TYPE Singletrack   **TOTAL ASCENT** 670 Feet

Nestled into a final hilly nook of the Taconics before they give way to the Champlain Valley Lowlands not far to the north, Vermont's newest state park features a terrific network of marked trails that visit dramatic cliff-top vistas, wide-open meadows, and secluded waterfalls in dark forest ravines. In essence, Taconic Mountains Ramble State Park offers exactly what its rambling name promises. The property includes a diverse mix of natural habitats and trail types as well as a manicured "Japanese Garden" setting, complete with miniature waterfalls, quaint footbridges, and tranquil waterside benches. The literal high point is 1,207-ft. Zion Hill (a.k.a. Mount Zion) and the low points cross small brooks between active hayfields. Primary trail loops are well marked, signed, and maintained, though some of the side trails are a bit rougher, wilder, and more primitive. The site, which is generally undeveloped as parks go, was donated in 2016 by former owners Carson "Kit" Davidson and his wife, Mickie.

DIRECTIONS   From Rte. 4, Exit 5 in Castleton, take E Hubbardton/ Monument Hill Road north for 6.2 miles. Turn left onto St. John Road and go 0.3 miles west. Turn left onto the access road for Taconic Mountains Ramble State Park and go 0.25 miles south up to the first parking lot (the main parking lot is another quarter mile up the road). **GPS:** "321 St. John Rd, Hubbardton, VT"

TRAIL   From the first parking lot, go south on the access road for 0.2 miles. Just before reaching an open field, go left into the woods on the yellow-blazed Mickie's North Woods Trail. Follow this wide,

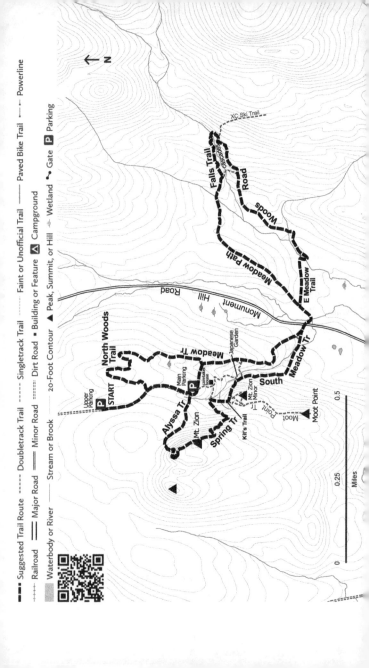

← N

Suggested Trail Route   Doubletrack Trail   Singletrack Trail   Faint or Unofficial Trail   Paved Bike Trail   Powerline
+++ Railroad   Major Road   Minor Road   Dirt Road   ▲ Campground
Waterbody or River   Stream or Brook   20-Foot Contour   ▲ Peak, Summit, or Hill   ⬥ Wetland   • Gate   P Parking

XC Ski Trail

Falls Trail

Road

Woods

Meadow Path

E Meadow Trail

Monument Hill Road

North Woods Trail

Meadow Tr

Japanese Garden

South Meadow Tr

Upper Parking

START

Main Parking

P

Alyssa Tr

Mt. Zion

Spring Tr

Kit's Trail

Mt. Zion Minor

Moot Point Tr

Moot Point

0   0.25   0.5

Miles

winding trail through the woods for 0.3 miles; the footing is rather rooty in places. When it arrives at an open field, the trail changes names to Meadow Trail. Follow the wide, mowed path of Meadow Trail south out in the open, passing a bench on the left and taking in the expansive views of the Taconic Mountains in the distance. In 0.25 miles, go right at a junction and follow the path west over to the main parking area (where there is an outhouse).

Cross the parking lot to the access road; the park manager home is on the left. Just a little bit north on the west side, look for the Alyssa Trail sign at the edge of the woods. After crossing a wooden bridge, follow Alyssa Trail west up through the rocky woods for 0.25 miles to the base of a talus slope of large boulders. Carefully climb up through the fern-covered rocks. At the base of the cliff, bear right and climb steeply up the side of the hill via stone steps, a wooden bridge, and narrow ledges to the top of Mount Zion Major where there are amazing views from the first open ledge.

Go south through a short, wooded dip to a second open ledge (the trail briefly changes names to Jan Trail here). Descend south on the white-blazed Spring Trail (with occasional red marker arrows at sharp turns), which switchbacks 0.2 miles down the hillside. At a junction, go right for 0.1 mile on the yellow-blazed Kit's Trail. Cross a bridge and go left at a junction where the Moot Point/Mount Zion Minor Trails lead right.

Optional Extension Take a right here to complete a short loop on the yellow-blazed Mount Zion Minor Trail and do an out-and-back on the Moot Point Trail to Moot Point (where there is another good vista). The ledgy descent from Mount Zion Minor is very steep and not recommended for running.

Follow the now white-blazed Kit's Trail 0.1 mile down past large boulders to the Japanese Garden, a manicured set of small pools flanked by large rocks where secured Adirondack chairs perch in surprising spots. On the other side of the garden, look for the sign pointing "to eastern trails." Follow the South Meadow Trail 0.1 mile south through the woods to the upper end of South Meadow. Then take the wide, mown path through the field 0.15 mile down to Monument Hill Road.

Carefully cross the road and follow the gravelly/grassy road, curving left and crossing a bridge. In 0.1 mile, go right at a junction to start onto the east side of Eastern Meadow Trail. Follow the wide, mown path to a stream crossing, then trace the left edge of another field. At another junction, go left on Woods Road.

Cross a stream and climb gradually on the white-blazed Woods Road for 0.25 miles, passing a short connector path on the left. There are occasional blue cross-country ski trail markers. At a junction, go left on Falls Trail and cross the stream at a metal cable. Descend Falls Trail on the other side for 0.1 mile, passing numerous scenic cascades in the steep-sided, rocky gorge on the left along the way (may be dry in summer). Bear right at a junction and continue 0.25 miles south on Falls Trail, which becomes Meadow Path at the edge of a field.

Follow the wide, mown path 0.3 miles up into and across a field, then down the other side of the hill to a junction. Follow the grassy road back to and across Monument Hill Road. At a junction, go right and ascend Meadow Trail for 0.25 miles along the left edge of an open field. Go left at the path to the main parking area, then follow the access road back to the upper parking lot; there may be a mown path beside the road.

NEARBY There's a surprising lack of official trails in the hills on either side of the east-west Rte. 4 corridor through the northern Taconics, with a few notable exceptions. About ten miles to the southeast of the park, the 1.2-mile Whipple Hollow Trail traverses **West Rutland Marsh** at the eastern base of **Hanley Mountain**.

DISTANCE 4.5 Miles   **TOWN** Rutland

DIFFICULTY RATING Moderate   **TRAIL STYLE** Loop

TRAIL TYPE Singletrack   **TOTAL ASCENT** 450 Feet

Nestled into the hillside northwest of Rutland, the city's forested Pine Hill Park boasts one of the finest community trail networks anywhere. There are singletrack trails for every skill level and all trails are well marked, well maintained, and fun to run. The suggested route here makes a relatively easy-to-follow loop through the park that showcases many of its attractions. Major junctions are marked with unique letters, and maps are posted at many of them. Terrain highlights include Rocky Pond, several scenic vistas, and glacial erratic boulders, and there are even occasional remote benches. The trail construction of some routes is truly outstanding, and several of the impressive wooden bridges in the park make worthy destinations in their own right. While most of the trails are multi-use—for mountain bikers, hikers, geocachers, and runners—several of the lower trails near the parking lot are for pedestrian use only; these loops make excellent routes for first-time trail runners or anyone looking for fewer interactions with other users.

DIRECTIONS   From Rte. 7 in Rutland, go 1 mile west on Crescent Street. Turn right on Preville Ave (one-way) and go 0.1 mile north then bear left on Oak Street Ext. Turn right into the parking lot for Giorgetti Athletic Complex and park in the designated area.

GPS: "Pine Hill Park, Rutland"

TRAIL   From the trailhead at the upper end of the parking lot, head west up the hill on the wide gravel path, curving right and passing the park sign and then bearing left at a bench by a map kiosk. Descend slightly

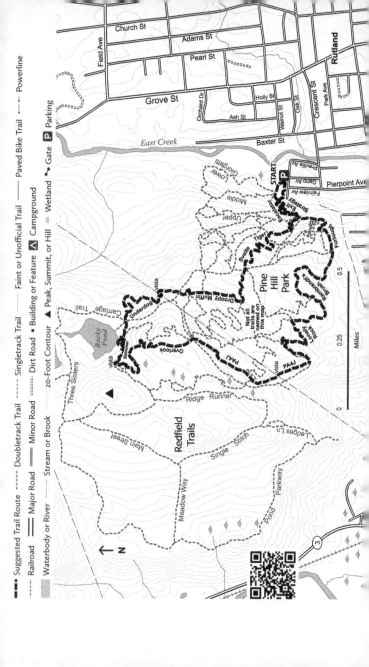

and cross a small marshy area on boardwalks. At a 5-way intersection by a boulder (this is junction 1; the pedestrian-only Giorgetti trails are to the right), bear left onto Escalator trail. Climb the gentle switchbacks of Escalator for 0.2 miles to a complicated intersection (9) just past some powerlines.

Go straight at the intersection, following signs for "Svelte Tiger" and "Rocky Pond 2.3 miles." Follow Svelte Tiger as it gently winds up the hill for 0.5 miles (see figure 4). At a junction (17), cross Trillium Trail and continue climbing on Svelte Tiger. In a short distance, cross the elaborate Sleeping Ledge Bridge over a rocky wet area.

In 0.3 miles, at jct. 22, cross Watkins Wood Road and begin climbing Droopy Muffin, again at a gentle grade. In 0.15 miles, bear right at jct. 22A, then straight at jct. 26 in another 0.15 miles. Shortly after, take a right onto Underdog at jct. 26A. Follow Underdog for 0.5 miles to a junction (32) near Rocky Pond. Along the way you'll re-cross Watkins Wood Road, cross an open powerline swath with a bench and a view, and traverse the banked Centrifuge Bridge (being mindful of bikes). The trail braids several times at marked forks.

At jct. 32, go straight onto Shimmer. In 0.1 mile, cross 999 trail at jct. 31 and immediately go over the fairytale-like Arch Bridge. Then follow Shimmer as it switchbacks up above the south shore of Rocky Pond to a magnificent northeast vista at the Overlook ledges (jct. 31); be careful of deep cracks in the rocks at the vista. This clearing makes a great picnic spot.

Go south on Overlook, bearing left at a braid fork to take the Lichen Rock option. Follow Overlook south for 0.5 miles, crossing a bouncy wooden suspension bridge along the way.

At jct. 30, follow the sign for "Trailhead via Lonely Rock 2.3 mi." and take the PA4J trail southwest at a very gentle downhill grade for 0.3 miles. Go straight at jct. 34 to stay on PA4J, which you'll follow for another 0.25 miles. Cross a powerline and arrive at jct. 28, where a sign says, "Trailhead 1.5 mi." Go left onto Lonely Rock and follow it for 0.6 miles to jct. 25, staying right at a fork, jct. 28A, and jct. 25A.

From jct. 25, go straight on Rembrandt's Brush and follow it downhill for 0.4 miles to jct. 20. Go straight and follow Furlough downhill for 0.3 miles to jct. 9. Take the one-way Exit Strategy trail 0.25 miles downhill back to the trailhead.

Optional Extensions Options for extending the loop are endless, ranging from adding in extra interior trail loops to venturing west onto Redfield Trails or heading north on Carriage Trail.

NEARBY From Rocky Pond, the wide **Carriage Trail** extends another four miles north to Proctor. Bordering Pine Hill Park to the west, the **Redfield Trails** network features a number of wide loops; major junctions are marked with letters. A few miles north, Pittsford's 2.3-mile **Cadwell Trail** loop makes an easy, flat circuit through mown fields and along Otter Creek.

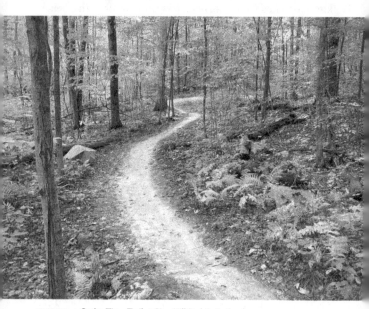

FIGURE 4. Svelte Tiger Trail at Pine Hill Park in Rutland.

DISTANCE 12 Miles   **TOWN** Poultney

DIFFICULTY RATING Moderate   **TRAIL STYLE** Figure-8 Loop

TRAIL TYPE Singletrack   **TOTAL ASCENT** 1,470 Feet

The wonderful Slate Valley Trails (SVT) network encompasses a huge, mostly interconnected number of singletrack and doubletrack trails in the low, rolling Taconic hills east of Poultney. The two primary trail systems are called Fairgrounds and Endless Brook. This suggested route roughly follows the course of an annual half-marathon race at the Fairgrounds system, but fun, scenic loops can be launched from any of the trailheads. Extension possibilities are seemingly limitless on the many connecting trails of the SVT network. Note that these trails are entirely on private property and open to the public only through the landowner's generosity and partnership with SVT; please take extra care to respect all posted rules and guidelines.

DIRECTIONS   from Poultney, take Rte. 140 east for 3.8 miles. Bear left onto Town Farm Road and go 0.1 mile up to the gravel parking lot on the right, across from a mountain-bike pumptrack loop. If the designated lot is full, there is overflow parking in the field next to the red barn. **GPS:** "Slate Valley Trails, 131 Town Farm Road, Poultney"

TRAIL   from the Fairgrounds trailhead, head northwest down the hill on Parking Lot Connector, the curvy gravel path paralleling Town Farm Road. In 0.1 mile, cross the road and pass between fence posts to the dirt road beyond. Go right and ascend gradually on Sugar Maple for 0.2 miles on the dirt road.

At an intersection, go left and drop 0.1 mile down to Rte. 140. Carefully cross the road and follow the wide Ringmaster trail 0.2 miles to a junction. Take a right on the singletrack Cotton Candy

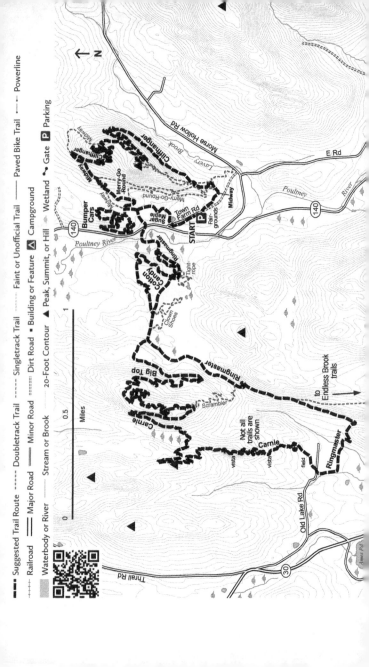

trail and follow it 0.8 twisty but gentle miles back to a junction with Ringmaster, skirting the edges of several open fields along the way. Cross Ringmaster and follow Clown Shoes, another winding single-track trail for 0.5 miles back to another junction with Ringmaster. Go left on Ringmaster and follow it several hundred feet west to a junction.

Take a right on Big Top and follow it for 2.3 circuitous miles as it meanders up and down the wooded hillside at gentle grades with excellent footing, passing several ledge-top vistas along the way. At a junction with Scrambler (which drops back down to Ringmaster), take a right on Carnie and follow it northwest across the slope, then down to and across a wetland, and up the slope of another hill. In 1.6 miles there is a view from the top of the hill. From here, drop down Carnie for 0.7 intensely curvy, switchback-filled miles to Old Lake Road, passing in and out of a hillside meadow with splendid views of the bucolic valley below along the way.

Cross the road and follow Ringmaster south into a field, then east past a pond and up the lower slopes of a forested hill. In 0.8 miles, reach a junction with the connector trail from Endless Brook which comes in from the south. Go straight and follow Ringmaster northeast for 2 easy miles back to the junction with Sugar Maple in the field east of Rte. 140. Take a left and go 0.1 mile north to a 4-way intersection.

Optional Extension For a fun, easy to moderate 1-mile lollipop loop on banked singletrack, go left and follow the Bumper Cars trail in either direction as it swoops around the hillside.

Take a right at the intersection and follow Merry-Go-Round 0.1 mile uphill through the field to a junction where the trail starts a loop. Go left and follow Merry-Go-Round 0.1 mile across the field to an upper junction with Midway. Bear right and follow Merry-Go-Round uphill into the woods for 0.15 miles; it criss-crosses back and forth over the wide but steep Midway trail several times. At the uppermost intersection of the two, go left on Midway and follow it for 0.2 miles to a junction.

Go right and follow Cliffhanger trail as it switchbacks 0.7 miles up the side of the steep hill; this section of trail is technical and challenging. From the top, follow Cliffhanger 1.4 miles down the hill to a junction near the bottom, passing alternate options like Freefall and Loop-the-Loop trails along the way. Bear left and follow Midway trail 0.1 mile southwest to the trailhead.

NEARBY One mile to the northwest, two loops combine for about 3 miles of trail at **Howe Hill** in East Poultney. A few miles west, the mostly flat, 3.3-mile multi-use **Poultney River and Rail Trail (PRRT)** rings downtown Poultney; in addition to the dirt hiking trail part along the river, it includes portions of the D&H Rail Trail as well as several paved road sections. Parking is at Bentley Avenue in Poultney. Just south of SVT's **Endless Brook** trail system, the combined Yellow (steep) and Green (gentler) trails at the pedestrian-only **Lewis Deane Nature Preserve** form a nice, moderately difficult 1.9-mile loop with terrific views of Lake St. Catherine. Further southwest, there are about 5 miles of non-motorized trails at **Delaney Woods** in Wells.

DISTANCE 7 Miles   **TOWN** Mount Tabor
DIFFICULTY RATING Moderate   **TRAIL STYLE** Loop
TRAIL TYPE Singletrack   **TOTAL ASCENT** 1,217 Feet

The terrific Green Mountain–Little Rock Pond loop feels somewhat like a greatest hits tour of the Green Mountains of Vermont, with several varieties of forest type, a conifer-covered peak with mossy green understory, scenic vistas on rocky ledges, a remote pond with an island, and even a stretch of the famous Long Trail/Appalachian Trail (LT/AT). There are several spots along the shore of Little Rock Pond where you can cool off with a swim. The rugged, mountain portion of this loop is much less frequently traveled than the popular Little Rock Pond part. Though the footing is generally good the whole way, the usual rocks and roots are common and several short pitches over rocky ledges on the north side of Green Mountain are very steep. The entire route falls within the Green Mountain National Forest.

DIRECTIONS From Rte. 7 in Danby, take Brooklyn Road (Forest Road 10) east up through Mount Tabor for 3.5 miles to the LT/AT crossing. The parking area is on the south side of the road.
GPS: "USFS 10 Big Branch Parking Area"

TRAIL From the parking lot, turn left on FR10 and go west. In 100 feet, just after crossing over a brook, enter the woods on the blue-blazed Green Mountain Connector Trail on the right. Follow this trail 0.7 miles southwest as it rises and falls through northern hardwood forest along the lower slopes of Green Mountain. At a junction with Green Mountain Trail, take a right (to the left, this trail drops steeply down to the Big Branch overlook and picnic area on Brooklyn Road).

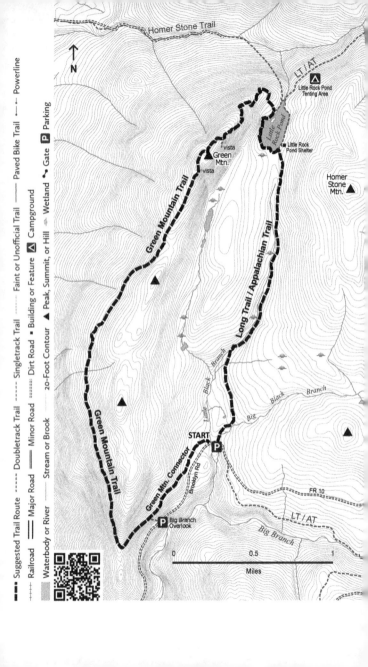

Legend:

- ■■■ Suggested Trail Route
- ┅┅┅ Doubletrack Trail
- ----- Faint or Unofficial Trail
- ━━━ Paved Bike Trail
- ┼┼┼ Railroad
- ━━━ Major Road
- ----- Singletrack Trail
- ┉┉┉ Minor Road
- ┄┄┄ Dirt Road
- ━━━ Stream or Brook
- ━━━ 20-Foot Contour
- ■ Building or Feature
- ▲ Campground
- ▲ Peak, Summit, or Hill
- •⌇ Wetland
- •— Gate
- ↤┄ Powerline
- Waterbody or River
- 🅿 Parking

N ↑

Homer Stone Trail

LT / AT

Little Rock Pond Tenting Area

Little Rock Pond

vista
Green Mtn.
vista

Little Rock Pond Shelter

Homer Stone Mtn. ▲

Green Mountain Trail

Long Trail / Appalachian Trail

▲

▲

Little Black Branch

Black Branch

Big Branch

▲

START
🅿

▲

Green Mountain Trail

Green Mtn. Connector

Brooklyn Rd

FR 10

LT / AT

🅿 Big Branch Overlook

Big Branch

0   0.5   1

Miles

Begin climbing the blue-blazed Green Mountain Trail, steeply at first and then more gradually across a hemlock covered slope. In 0.25 miles it curves sharply right around the ridge at a small grassy patch with limited views west and then starts climbing north through hemlock–pine and mixed hardwood forest up the west side of the mountain at a moderate grade. The trail occasionally dips and descends slightly, but overall it continues to climb along the path of an old woods road for the next 2 miles. When it reaches the crest of the ridge the forest type changes to boreal spruce-fir and the mossy green understory really stands out.

Continue climbing north along the ridgecrest at a steady grade. At 3.2 miles from the start, a short spur path leads right to a limited vista of Peru Peak Wilderness to the east. Continue north on the soft, verdant trail along the ridge just west of the wooded 2,471-ft. summit for 0.25 miles to a junction. Take a right at a sign saying, "pond view" and follow the spur path south for several hundred feet down to an open rock outcrop with views.

From the junction, follow Green Mountain Trail 0.7 miles down to Little Rock Pond. Overall the grade is moderate but there are several very steep ledge drops. At one point the trail bypasses a cool-looking, narrow fin of ledge that the old trail used to go over.

Go right on Little Rock Pond Loop Trail and follow it south for 0.25 miles above the edge of the pond to a large ledge with a steep drop (see figure 5). Carefully descend the trail on the other side of the ledge and go 0.25 miles around the rooty south shore of the pond to a junction with the Long Trail/Appalachian Trail (LT/AT). From here it is 0.1 mile north to Little Rock Pond Shelter, built in 2010 near the site of the former Lula Tye Shelter (which was actually originally constructed on the island in the pond in 1962 and reached by a bridge until 1972).

To complete the loop, take a right and follow the white-blazed LT/AT south for 2.2 miles to the trailhead. After a short rise away from the pond, the trail drops steadily down a long stretch of boardwalk puncheon and past a number of small, open wetlands. It also crosses

Little Black Branch brook several times, including once on a narrow metal I-beam, before reaching the Big Black Branch parking lot.

NEARBY From this parking lot, it's a relatively easy 4.5-mile climb south on the **Long Trail** to the ledges on **Baker Peak**, or a 13.2-mile lollipop loop can be made by continuing on to **Griffith Lake** and returning via **Old Job Trail**. Several miles to the north, two short but scenic trails at **White Rocks National Recreation Area** are very much worth visiting: the 3.2-mile round-trip **White Rocks Cliffs Trail** and the 1.8-mile round-trip **Ice Beds Trail**.

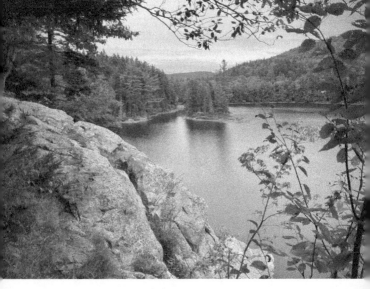

FIGURE 5. Little Rock Pond in Wallingford.

DISTANCE 8 Miles   **TOWN** Danby

DIFFICULTY RATING Moderate   **TRAIL STYLE** Lollipop Loop

TRAIL TYPE Singletrack   **TOTAL ASCENT** 2,175 Feet

This scenic lollipop loop route features a dramatic cliffside bridge, a remote mountain pond, and spectacular views from the exposed ledges of Baker peak. It incorporates a sustained, steady climb up from the valley into the Green Mountains with a section of the Long Trail/Appalachian Trail (LT/AT) in the Big Branch Wilderness Area, as well as a visit to Griffith Lake and a short out-and-back spur up steep, narrow ledges. There are occasional rocky, rooty, and muddy areas throughout, but overall the grade is generally moderate and the footing is good.

DIRECTIONS   From Mount Tabor, take Rte. 7 south for 2.5 miles. Turn left/east onto South End Road and go 0.5 miles to the parking pull-off on the left, just past a small brown National Forest hiker sign saying, "Lake Trailhead."

GPS: "Griffith Lake Trailhead"

TRAIL   The Lake Trail path enters the woods through a shrub thicket on the right side of the parking area. Follow the blue-blazed Lake Trail southeast at a gentle grade above a small stream. At 0.2 miles, dip down to cross the stream on rocks then continue climbing along the other side. At 0.7 miles, curve left and begin climbing up out of the valley at a steady, moderate grade along the track of a former bridle path. At 0.9 miles in, pass the Big Branch Wilderness sign.

At about 1.5 miles, the trail crosses the face of a sloping ledge on a wooden bridge with a metal railing. At 1.7 miles, the trail curves right and heads east up into a narrow stream valley, hugging the steep

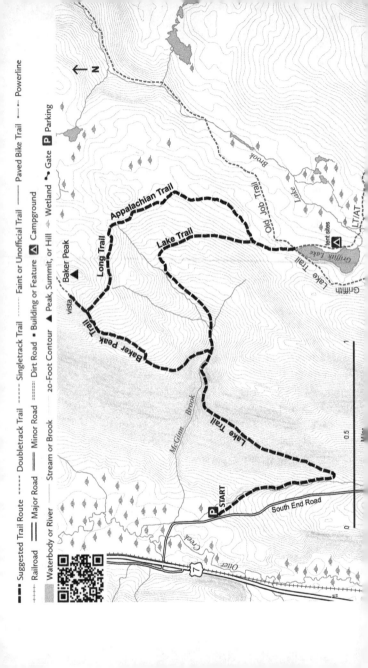

slope above McGinn Brook. After passing some cascades, cross the stream on rocks (which may be difficult during high water) and reach a junction at 1.9 miles up from the trailhead.

Begin the loop part of the route by going straight ahead and following the still blue-blazed Lake Trail east along the north side of the stream. Cross over it in a few hundred feet and then continue gradually climbing east through hardwoods. In 0.5 miles, bear east away from a wetland and climb south for 0.5 miles to a junction.

Go straight and follow the white-blazed LT/AT 0.25 miles south down to the northern shore of Griffith Lake. To reach the water's edge, go right for a short distance on an unmarked woods road (see

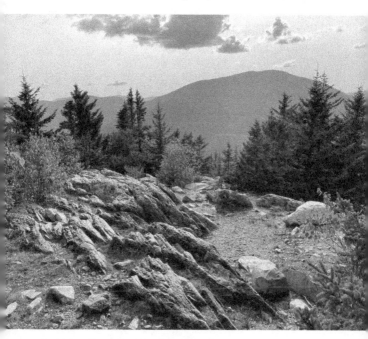

FIGURE 6. View of Dorset Peak from ledges on Baker Peak.

site 7 for more details about the trails around the lake). Then head north back to the junction, take a right and follow the LT/AT north/northwest over rolling terrain for 1.6 miles to a junction.

Take a right and scramble up the LT/AT on the rugged ledges of Baker Peak. These exposed, narrow fins of rock—partly framed by stunted trees—feature excellent, expansive views west and southwest over Vermont Valley (see figure 6), though they can be very slippery when wet. There is also a little-used, roughly parallel Bad Weather Bypass trail that skirts around the ledges to the east. The actual, wooded summit of Baker Peak is off-trail.

From the ledges, carefully drop back to the junction and then go straight to descend the blue-blazed Baker Peak Trail, steeply at first then at a moderate grade, for 0.8 miles to the junction with Lake Trail. To complete the route, go right and follow Lake Trail back down to the trailhead.

NEARBY Just a few miles south on Rte. 7, the 2.6-mile Vista Trail at **Emerald Lake State Park** in North Dorset makes a moderately difficult lollipop loop along the forested, west-facing side of a lower sub-ridge of the Green Mountains escarpment above the lake and floor of the Vermont Valley. There is also a short trail along the west side of the lake.

DISTANCE 9.6 Miles   **TOWN** Danby

DIFFICULTY RATING Moderate   **TRAIL STYLE** Loop

TRAIL TYPE Singletrack   **TOTAL ASCENT** 1,740 Feet

This classic, roughly ten-mile trail run loop incorporates the Long Trail/Appalachian Trail (LT/AT), two high-elevation Green Mountain peaks (both above 3,000 feet), Griffith Lake, and a remote forest service fire road. While not quite as scenic overall as several other nearby loops, it nevertheless provides a satisfying workout in the wilderness, features relatively moderate grades when climbing, and includes an opportunity to cool off in the water partway through.

DIRECTIONS   From Main Street in Peru (off Rte. 11), take Hapgood Pond Road north for 1 mile. Bear left onto North Road and go 0.8 miles north. Turn left on Mad Tom Notch Road (Forest Road 21) and go 2.1 miles west to the parking area on the left.

GPS: "Long Trail Mad Tom Notch"

TRAIL   From the trailhead on the north side of the road, follow the white-blazed LT/AT north into the woods. The grade is gradual at first, then becomes steeper, and the footing becomes somewhat rocky as you climb into spruce-fir forest near the top. In 1.4 miles you will reach the 3,373-ft. summit of Styles Peak where there is a lookout with an excellent view.

From Styles Peak, descend briefly and follow the LT/AT north along the ridge for 1.7 miles, crossing several knobs and many boardwalks along the way, to the forested summit of 3,416-ft. Peru Peak. Descend steeply down through mossy woods on the north side of Peru Peak for 0.2 miles. The trail then bears west and the grade becomes more

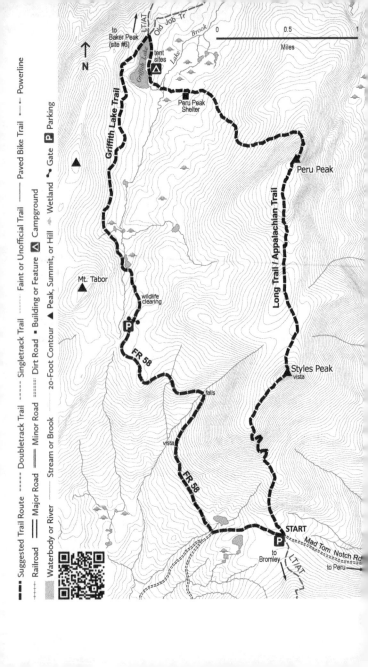

moderate. At 1.3 miles from the top, as the grade lessens even more, you will reach Peru Peak Shelter.

Drop down to a stream, cross it and then several others soon afterwards on wooden bridges, then climb 0.1 mile up to the southeastern side of Griffith Lake and cross a number of boardwalks over a wet area. Go north for 0.25 miles along the east side of the lake, passing a tenting area and crossing a long stretch of boardwalks to an intersection with Old Job Trail and Griffith Lake Trail.

Go left and follow the wide, unmarked Griffith Lake Trail (also a well-used snowmobile corridor) south along the west shore of the pond and then along the east side of a ridge for about 2 miles to a gated trailhead at the end of Forest Road 58. Continue south on Forest Road 58 for about 2 miles, descending most of the way, until you reach Mad Tom Notch Road. Then turn left and go east for about 0.5 miles back to the height of land at Mad Tom Notch, following (very) occasional blue blazes on the side of Mad Tom Notch Road.

NEARBY There are very few developed trails in the Peru Peak Wilderness Area. However, just south of this suggested route it is possible to make another very enjoyable 10-mile run by combining the LT/AT over **Bromley Mountain**, VAST snowmobile corridor 7, and Mad Tom Notch Road into a moderately challenging figure-8 loop.

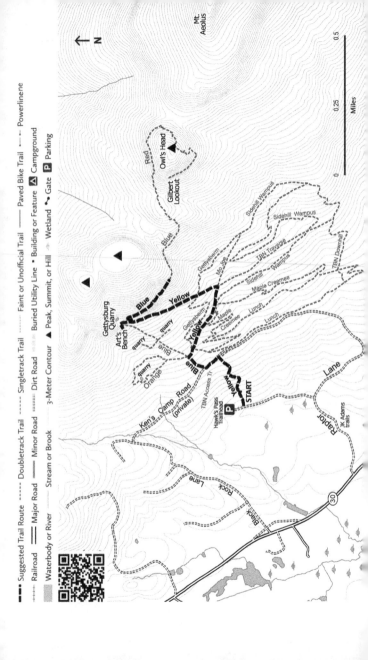

Suggested Trail Route ----- Doubletrack Trail ······· Singletrack Trail ----- Faint or Unofficial Trail ───── Paved Bike Trail ─ ── Powerlinene
++++ Railroad ══ Major Road ═════ Minor Road ═════ Dirt Road ····· Buried Utility Line · Building or Feature △ Campground
▓ Waterbody or River ── Stream or Brook ── 3-Meter Contour ▲ Peak, Summit, or Hill ◈ Wetland ⚬ Gate Ⓟ Parking

← N

Mt. Aeolus

Owl's Head

Red

Gilbert Lookout

Blue

Blue   Yellow

Gettysburg Quarry

Art's Bench

quarry   quarry

Blue

quarry   Orange

Gettysburg

Yellow

Yellow

Blue

Yellow

START

Ⓟ

Hawk's Pass Trailhood

TBN Access Tr

Ken's Camp Road (private)

Gettyberm

Mo Joe

Maple Creemee

Maple Creemee

Sidehill Wampus

Sidehill Wampus

TBN Traverse

Sidehill

Wampus

Maple Creemee

Lunch

Lunch

TBN Downhill

Lane

Raptor

JK Adams trails

Black

Rock   Lane

30

0   0.25   0.5

Miles

8   Owl's Head

DISTANCE 2.8 Miles (5 with extension to lookout)   **TOWN** Dorset

DIFFICULTY RATING Moderate   **TRAIL STYLE** Out-and-Back

TRAIL TYPE Singletrack   **TOTAL ASCENT** 675 Feet (1,500 Feet with extension to lookout)

Owl's Head Town Forest and adjacent properties host a network of marked hiking and biking trails on the south side of 2,474-ft. Owl's Head Peak. This suggested route visits several old quarries and scenic vistas; a more challenging optional extension goes up to a precipitous lookout ledge on Owl's Head itself. Note that for safety reasons the forest is closed to hikers, runners, and mountain bikers during parts of the late fall season.

DIRECTIONS From Manchester Center, take Rte. 30 north for 4.4 miles towards Dorset, then take a right on Raptor Lane. Go 0.3 miles up Raptor Lane, then take a left at a sign for the Owl's Head Town Forest trailhead. The small parking lot is 0.3 miles north up at the end of this unnamed dirt road.

GPS: "Raptor Lane, Dorset" (then follow signs to trailhead)

TRAIL From the parking area, go back down the dirt road a few hundred feet to the trailhead. At the map kiosk, cross the small wooden bridge and enter the woods to the north. Follow the trail, blazed with yellow diamond markers, as it switchbacks steadily up the hillside for 0.25 miles. Cross a mountain-bike trail and then take a left on Raptor Lane. Go 0.1 mile west down the wide dirt road to the old parking area at a cul-de-sac.

Take the wide trail just left of the Owl's Head Town Forest map kiosk and begin heading north up the hill, following blue and yellow diamond markers. In 0.1 mile, you will come to a junction with a trail on the right.

Optional Extension(s) From this junction, you can add an easy 0.6-mile extension by continuing up the hill a few hundred feet then bearing left on the Lower Prince Quarry Loop Trail. Follow this lollipop loop, marked with orange diamonds, as it traces an oval below and above an old quarry. This extension can be lengthened to 1.1 miles by adding in out-and-back spurs to Klondike Quarry and Middle Prince Quarry, each one branching off from the blue diamond trail several hundred feet above.

Go right on the yellow diamond trail and ascend the hillside at a steady, moderate grade, crossing or passing several mountain-bike trail junctions along the way. Following the yellow markers, take a left at the intersection that is currently marked with a 2-foot-high, plastic saluting Santa Claus, and continue following the yellow diamond trail west up the slope. At a junction, continue straight ahead for 0.1 mile to Gettysburg Quarry.

At Gettysburg Quarry, go left on a short spur trail over to a marble slab called "Art's Bench" at a vista with a great view looking southwest over Dorset towards Mother Myrick Mountain and Spruce Peak on the other side of the valley. The quarry itself can also be approached by a short spur path that ends at a pool in front of the old mine.

From the junction below the quarry, go up a set of stone steps and follow the blue-diamond-marked trail as it first switchbacks up the hill and then traverses the slope, climbing at a steady southeasterly grade. At about 0.25 miles up from the junction you will come to a clearing, where the trail crosses the upper part of a small open ledge, with a panoramic view to the south. From the vista, return back the way you came to complete the 3-mile route.

Optional Extension From the vista, continue east up the trail for 1.1 more miles to Gilbert Lookout. This trail becomes progressively steeper and more technical as it goes, and the final overhanging ledge can be quite dangerous so it is not recommended for children or anyone afraid of heights. After leaving the vista, the rise is gradual at first, then steeper as the trail switchbacks up towards Owl's Head Peak. When the blazes change color to red, the trail circles nearly halfway around the peak on a narrow, rocky, technical trail before going over it and starting down the other side. Finally, it bears right, levels out, and traverses west on the south side of the peak to Gilbert Lookout, a small ledge with a view. Look for a "Gilbert Lookout" rock plaque attached to a ledge outcrop nearby. Note that the old connector trail is permanently closed due to erosion.

NEARBY The bike trail network below the quarries is primarily designed for bikes but can be used with care by pedestrians, yielding to bikers when necessary; note that some of these trails are marked "one-way" only. A few miles north, a steep and rugged trail climbs 3,770-ft. **Dorset Mountain** from a trailhead at the upper end of Tower Road. A few miles east, woods roads and overgrown trails can be followed from Dorset Hill Road up the east side of 3,209-ft. **Mount Aeolus**, passing numerous old quarries and vistas along the way. Note that while portions of the old horseshoe-shaped Dorset Trail—which was built in the 1920s and visited many of the high Taconic peaks of the Dorset Uplift north and east of Dorset—have been revived and are in current use, many sections are no longer maintained or open to the public.

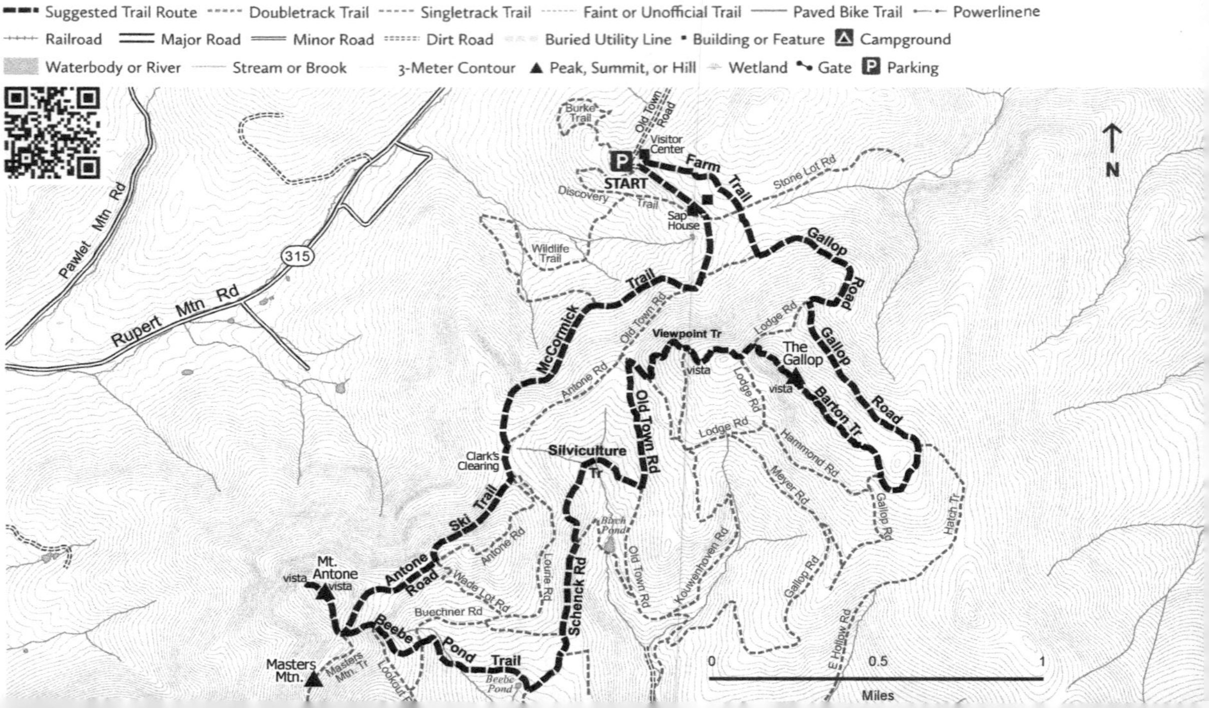
Suggested Trail Route
Doubletrack Trail
Singletrack Trail
Faint or Unofficial Trail
Paved Bike Trail
Powerlinene
Railroad
Major Road
Minor Road
Dirt Road
Buried Utility Line
Building or Feature
Campground
Waterbody or River
Stream or Brook
3-Meter Contour
Peak, Summit, or Hill
Wetland
Gate
Parking
N
Pawlet Mtn Rd
315
Rupert Mtn Rd
Burke Trail
Old Town Road
Visitor Center
START
Farm Trail
Discovery Trail
Stone Lot Rd
Sap House
Wildlife Trail
Gallop Road
McCormick Trail
Old Town Rd
Viewpoint Tr
Lodge Rd
The Gallop
vista
Barton Tr
Antone Rd
Old Town Rd
Hammond Rd
Meyer Rd
Clark's Clearing
Silviculture Tr
Ski Trail
Birch Pond
Kouwenhoven Rd
Gallop Rd
Hatch Tr
Lourie Rd
Mt. Antone
Antone Road
Wade Lot Rd
Schenck Rd
Buechner Rd
Beebe Pond Trail
Masters Mtn.
Masters Mtn. Tr
Beebe Pond
E Hollow Rd
0
0.5
1
Miles

DISTANCE 8 Miles   **TOWN** Rupert

DIFFICULTY RATING Moderate   **TRAIL STYLE** Loop

TRAIL TYPE Singletrack/Doubletrack   **TOTAL ASCENT** 1,460 Feet

The 30-mile Merck Forest trail system is one of the region's finest outdoor recreation gems. Covering a conservation area of over 2,800 acres, the network includes everything from wide woods roads to narrow hiking and cross-country ski trails. Trails visit the summits of several notable peaks, including Mount Antone, Masters Mountain, and Gallop Peak/Spruce Peak. There are numerous rustic backcountry cabins available to rent on site, as well as a public visitor center, working farm, and maple sugar production facility. The trails are very well marked and maintained, and trail maps are posted at many intersections. The grounds and trails are open to the public for free year-round from dawn to dusk.

DIRECTIONS   From Dorset, take Rte. 30 northwest for 2 miles. Take a left on Rte. 315 and go 2.6 miles west. Turn left on Merck Forest access road and go 0.5 miles up to the large dirt parking lot below the Visitor Center.

GPS: "Merck Forest & Farmland Center" or "3270 Rte. 315, Rupert"

TRAIL   From the Visitor Center, follow the dirt access road (Old Town Road) 0.25 miles southeast up the hill. After coming out into an open field and passing the caretaker's house on the left and the Sap House on the right you'll arrive at an intersection. Go straight and follow Old Town Road south gently down and then up alongside a field. In 0.2 miles, stay straight at a junction with Gallop Road. In a few hundred feet, just after the road enters the woods and curves right, take a right at a junction.

Follow the doubletrack-width McCormick Trail down the slope and past a junction with Wildlife Trail. At about 0.4 miles, begin climbing diagonally southwest up the hillside at a steady, moderate grade. In 0.6 miles, take a right on the wide Antone Road, then in 0.1 mile reach an intersection just past the cabin beyond Clark's Clearing.

Go right on Antone Ski Trail and again climb diagonally up the hillside at a steady, moderate grade for 0.4 miles to an upper junction with Antone Road. Go right on Antone Road, and follow it 0.4 miles up to an intersection in a saddle, passing junctions with Wade Lot Road and Lookout Road on the left. Take a hard right and follow the rough, rocky road steeply for 0.2 miles up to the 2,600-ft. top of Antone Mountain. Cross over the summit to a north-facing trailside vista just beyond, then drop 0.1 mile down to a spectacular, wide-open vista from a sub-peak on the mountain's west ridge.

Return to the junction in the saddle 0.2 miles below the summit. Take the narrow, zig-zaggy Beebe Pond Trail steeply downslope to the east for 0.8 miles to Beebe Pond shelters, crossing the wider Lookout Road and Buechner Trail along the way.

From Beebe Pond, take the wide Wade Lot Road 0.2 miles north up to a junction with Schenck Road. Go right on Schenck Road and gently descend 0.4 miles to a junction. Go left on the narrow Silviculture Trail and follow for 0.5 miles as it curves to the northeast around a forest cove and rises gently to a junction. Go left on the wide Old Town Road and climb gently for 0.2 miles to a junction just past a field on the right.

Take a sharp right on the wide Lodge Road. In 0.1 mile, take a left onto the narrow Viewpoint Trail and follow it as it switchbacks 0.25 miles up the hillside, steeply at times, to a junction. Go left on Viewpoint Road and climb 0.1 mile in the open to Viewpoint Cabin, where, as the name implies, there is a magnificent view.

From the cabin, take the Spur to Lodge Road path 0.2 miles through the woods and up to Lodge Road and take a left. Go 0.1 mile northeast on Lodge Road, then take a right on the narrow Barton Trail. Ascend the narrow Barton Trail at a *very* steep grade for 0.2 miles up to the ridgecrest of The Gallop (2,585 feet). This mountain was formerly called Spruce Peak, as seen on some older maps. The trail undulates along and then down the ridge for 0.4 miles to a junction with Gallop Road. Go left and follow Gallop Road up and around the east side of the ridge, pass a junction with the upper end of Hatch Trail, then gradually descend 0.4 miles to a junction with Lodge Road (this last section tends to get a bit seepy and muddy in places).

Drop steeply down Gallop Road for 0.5 miles to a junction (rising slightly at the bottom just past a junction with the closed Marquand Road) before Barn Cabins. Take a right and follow an unmarked connector path 0.2 miles down past a fence through an open field to the farm. Cross Stone Lot Road at an intersection and follow Farm Trail 0.1 mile up to the edge of the woods. Bear left and follow Farm Trail 0.2 miles down to the Visitor Center.

Optional Extensions   There are many possible extensions to this route at Merck, and most are fun and worthwhile. Any that descend all the way down to Old Town Road in Hidden Valley to the south will require a long climb back up and over, but there are also numerous cabins, ponds, and lookouts that way; the sometimes-grassy and sometimes-rocky (but always wide) Masters Mountain Trail, which switchbacks at a gentle grade on the southwest side of that peak with decent footing the whole way, is particularly fun to run. Discovery Trail and Wildlife Trail make nice footpath loop options on the lower northern slopes near the Sap House.

NEARBY A few miles northwest, the **Delaware and Hudson Rail Trail** runs north–south just east of the NY–VT state line and connects the communities of West Pawlet and Rupert.

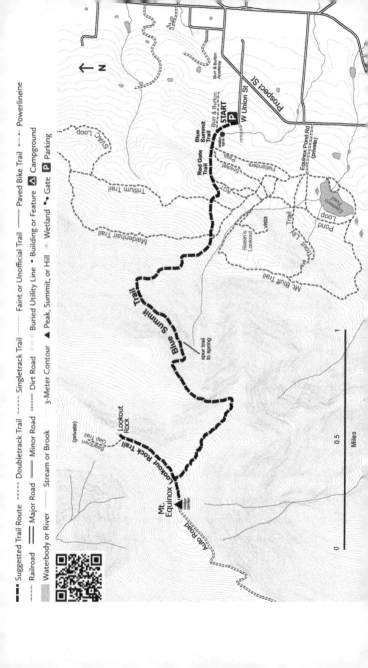

DISTANCE 6.2 Miles   **TOWN** Manchester

DIFFICULTY RATING Challenging   **TRAIL STYLE** Out-and-Back

TRAIL TYPE Singletrack   **TOTAL ASCENT** 2,840 Feet

Towering above the southwest side of Manchester, 3,825-ft. tall Mount Equinox is the highest peak in the entire Taconic Range. Upper trails on the mountain often retain snow well into the spring. The suggested route here is relentlessly steep for long stretches but includes panoramic views from the top as well as a spur path north to Lookout Rock. The new Visitor Center at the summit is privately owned and can also be accessed by an automobile toll road; it is often crowded and closes relatively early in the afternoon. Lower down on the east slope, a network of significantly gentler, multi-use trails loop around past ponds and through the woods. Most trail junctions are marked with wooden posts and trail names, and some also have maps. The trail network is maintained by The Equinox Preservation Trust and The Nature Conservancy while the St. Bruno's Scenic Viewing Center at the summit is maintained by the Carthusian Monks of Manchester, VT.

DIRECTIONS   From the rotary in Manchester Center, take Rte. 7A south for 1.1 miles. Bear right onto Seminary Avenue and go 0.3 miles southwest. Turn right and go 0.2 miles west on West Union Street. The small parking lot is on the right.

GPS: "Red Gate Trail W Union Street Manchester"

TRAIL   At the Red Gate trailhead, pass through the red metal gate and start uphill on the wide Red Gate trail (an old dirt road). In a few hundred feet, pass a water tower in a field on the left and a map kiosk on the right. Now follow red and blue blazes of the combined Red Gate and Blue Summit trails up into the woods of the Mount

Equinox Preserve for 0.1 mile to a junction with the blue-blazed Burr & Burton trail on the right. Bear left and go 0.1 mile west to junctions for Flatlanders and The Snicket trails in rapid succession on the left. The road surface starts to get rougher around here. Continue west up the hill for 0.2 miles to a fork where Red Gate trail veers left.

Bear right and follow Blue Summit Trail uphill at a slightly steeper grade through a parcel called Thompson Acres. In 0.15 miles, pass an intersection with Trillium Trail and a cabin in the woods on the left, then climb another 0.15 miles to an intersection with Maidenhair trail. Here you cross back onto Mount Equinox Preserve property.

Continue west upslope on the doubletrack-width Blue Summit Trail for 0.8 miles at a moderately steep grade. At a spruce thicket the trail abruptly narrows to singletrack, then soon reaches a junction next to a small wooden bench. Here, a short side trail leads south across the slope to a spring.

Bear right and continue upslope on the now significantly rougher and steeper Blue Summit Trail. It switches back and forth a few times and then climbs diagonally south up through mixed hardwood-conifer forest at a steady, steep grade. At 0.5 miles up from the spring path, it swings sharply right and begins a more moderate ascent through spruce-fir forest. Portions of this section may remain wet throughout the year. In 0.5 miles the trail arrives at a small clearing with a shed and then reaches a junction.

Take a left to climb gently for 0.1 mile on the Lookout Rock Trail to the Visitor Center at the summit, where there are expansive views in all directions. Descend back down to the junction and stay straight to descend at a gentle grade for 0.4 miles along the ridge on the Lookout Rock Trail, passing a stone bench and memorial gravestone for Mr. Barbo (a dog killed by a hunter in 1955), to a junction with Beartown Gap Trail. Bear right and rise 0.1 mile to a small vista overlooking Manchester at Lookout Rock, where there is another stone bench. To return to the trailhead, go back up to the junction, take a left and descend Blue Summit Trail the way you came.

Optional Extension(s) The network of trails on the lower slopes of Equinox provide a completely different type of trail-run experience. One relatively easy option is to make a ~2-mile loop to Equinox Pond by combining Flatlanders, Trillium, Pond Loop, and Red Gate trails. Longer, more moderately difficult loops could incorporate the white-blazed Mount Bluff trail or yellow-blazed Maidenhair trail.

NEARBY The 2.2-mile **Beartown Gap Trail** on the north side of Equinox offers gentler grades along an old road, though there is no official parking at the north end.

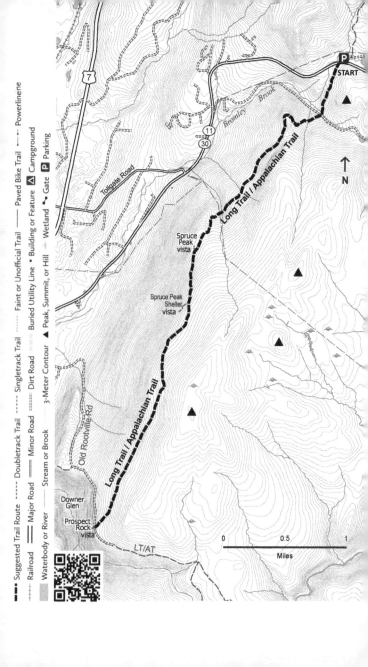

Suggested Trail Route ···· Doubletrack Trail ----- Singletrack Trail ----- Faint or Unofficial Trail ━━ Paved Bike Trail ⊢-⊣ Powerlinene
+++++ Railroad ══ Major Road ⁼⁼⁼ Minor Road ⁝⁝⁝⁝⁝ Dirt Road ⋯⋯ Buried Utility Line • Building or Feature ▲ Campground
〰 Waterbody or River — Stream or Brook — 3-Meter Contour ▲ Peak, Summit, or Hill ⧫ Wetland ⌐ Gate 🅿 Parking

7

Bromley Brook

🅿
START

▲

11
30

Tollgate Road

N

Long Trail / Appalachian Trail

Spruce
Peak
vista

▲

Spruce Peak
Shelter
vista

▲

Old Rootville Rd

Long Trail / Appalachian Trail

▲

Downer
Glen

Prospect
Rock
vista

LT/AT

0   0.5   1

Miles

DISTANCE 9.5 Miles   **TOWN** Winhall and Manchester

DIFFICULTY RATING Moderate   **TRAIL STYLE** Out-and-Back

TRAIL TYPE Singletrack   **TOTAL ASCENT** 1,790 Feet

This out-and-back section of the Long Trail/Appalachian Trail (LT/AT) runs along a stretch with no significantly prominent mountains. It is by no means level, however, as the trail constantly rises and falls along the upper edge of the Green Mountains escarpment above Manchester in the valley to the west. Passing primarily through mixed hardwood forest, the route features several short spur trails to scenic vistas as well as a hiker's hut, and the soaring view from Prospect Rock ledge at the southern end is particularly dramatic. As with many easily accessible parts of the LT/AT in Vermont, it is fairly heavily used during the summer, and the parking lot along Rte. 11/30 is used by snowmobilers in the winter. Extreme caution is required for the busy road crossing of Rte. 11/30 at the northern end.

DIRECTIONS   From the rotary in Manchester Center, take Rte. 11/30 east for 6 miles up to the large parking lot on the left.

GPS: "Bromley Mountain, Long Trail"

TRAIL   From the trailhead go south and immediately cross the very busy Rte. 11/30. Be extremely careful at this road crossing. Rapidly go straight across while looking both ways. On the other side, head up into the woods on the white-blazed LT/AT. After a short rise, the trail levels off and begins descending at an easy grade just above Bromley Brook.

In 0.4 miles, cross a small stream on a wooden bridge and then cross an abandoned road. The base of one of the old Snow Valley Ski Area's lifts is a short distance uphill on the old road. Continue south on the LT/AT, rising at a gentle then moderate grade for 0.4 miles through a small boulder field and then around and up a ridge to a grassy knob.

Drop slightly to a saddle, descend for 0.25 miles, then traverse the hillside at a relatively level grade for 0.6 miles. Cross a semi-open powerline swath and a small stream, then climb steadily for 0.4 miles at a moderate grade to a junction.

Go right/west on a 0.1-mile, blue-blazed spur path that briefly scrambles up a steep, rocky ledge to the conifer-clad top of 2,041-ft. Spruce Peak where there is a west-facing vista. Return to the junction.

Continue south on the LT/AT, descending slightly at first then rising steadily for 0.4 miles at a moderate grade to a junction. Go right and follow a spur path 0.2 miles down to Spruce Peak Shelter; there is a ledge with a limited westerly view just past the log cabin. Return to the junction.

Continue south on the LT/AT. From here, the trail rises and falls several more times as it traverses the west slope of the escarpment before beginning a lengthy but gradual descent. In 2 miles, drop down a set of stone steps and cross Old Rootville Road, then follow the spur path south about a hundred feet down to Prospect Rock, a bare ledge outcrop with a commanding view of steep-sided Downer Glen just ahead and the broader Vermont Valley to the west. From Prospect Rock, go back up to the junction at Old Rootville Road and return to the trailhead along the LT/AT the way you came to complete the route.

NEARBY North of the parking lot, take the LT/AT up **Bromley Mountain** for a 5.3-mile round-trip trek. The climbing is relatively gentle at first, then moderate with occasional steep pitches before emerging out onto an open ski trail near the top. Six miles northeast, there's a nice mile-long trail around **Hapgood Pond** in Peru that makes an easy and scenic introductory trail run for beginners (though there are some slippery roots).

DISTANCE 4.4 Miles   **TOWN** Manchester
DIFFICULTY RATING Moderate   **TRAIL STYLE** Out-and-Back
TRAIL TYPE Singletrack   **TOTAL ASCENT** 940 Feet

Lye Brook Falls is one of the tallest waterfalls in New England, located about halfway up the length of Lye Brook, a major tributary of the Batten Kill river. The blue-blazed Lye Brook Trail climbs diagonally along an old road up the side of a steep wilderness valley at a relatively moderate grade. The 125-ft. waterfall actually consists of a series of cascades and horsetails tumbling down multiple tiers of steep, bare rock ledges. This very popular hiking destination is best visited during the week or early in the morning when crowds tend to be smaller. Most of the site is located within Green Mountain National Forest's Lye Brook Wilderness Area.

DIRECTIONS   From Rte. 11 east of Manchester, take East Manchester Road south for 1.1 miles. Turn left on Glen Road and cross Bourne Brook. In 0.1 mile, bear right onto the dirt Lye Brook Falls Access Road, the start of which can be eroded and rough. Go 0.35 miles south to the parking area and trailhead.
GPS: "Lye Brook Falls Trailhead"

TRAIL   On the southeast side of the parking area, follow either of two wide, rocky paths for a hundred feet or so over to a map kiosk with information about Lye Brook Wilderness. Then follow the blue-blazed Lye Brook Trail a few hundred feet through a shrubby area and up into the woods. The footing is alternately rocky, rooty, and smooth.

Bear left when the trail approaches the north bank of Lye Brook near a hiker registration post, then follow the trail nearly due south for about a mile at a gradually steepening grade, crossing into Lye

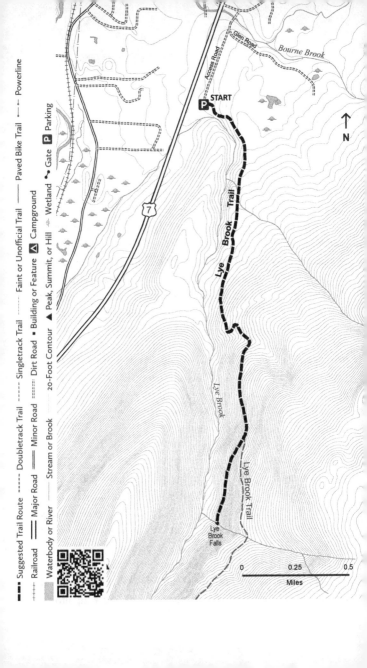

Legend

- ■■ Suggested Trail Route
- ---- Doubletrack Trail
- ----- Singletrack Trail
- ·········· Faint or Unofficial Trail
- —— Paved Bike Trail
- ← → Powerline
- +++ Railroad
- ═══ Major Road
- ═══ Minor Road
- ········ Dirt Road
- • Building or Feature
- ▲ Campground
- —— 20-Foot Contour
- ▲ Peak, Summit, or Hill
- —— Stream or Brook
- —— Waterbody or River
- ⟜ Wetland
- • Gate
- P Parking

START

Glen Road

Bourne Brook

Access Road

7

Lye Brook Trail

Lye Brook

Lye Brook Trail

Lye Brook Falls

N

0   0.25   0.5
Miles

Brook Wilderness along the way. At a curve to the left, go east up a switchback and then continue ascending south up the hillside for about half a mile to a junction, crossing several small streams along the way.

Bear right on the spur trail to the falls, which is narrower and marked with slightly lighter blue blazes. Descend slightly over roots and a few muddy sections, with the slope dropping away steeply on the right. Cross the open track of a narrow landslide scar, then continue through woods on the other side.

Once you can see the falls, stop running! The bluff is eroded and caution is required here. You can either drop steeply down a gravelly slope to the base of the falls or bear left to make your way along a narrow path below a cliff to ledges beside the middle of the falls. Return to the trailhead back the way you came.

Optional Extension Above the spur to the falls, the Lye Brook Trail continues up into the interior of the vast Lye Brook Wilderness. After several more miles of climbing, the grade levels out as the trail heads east across the plateau, where the trail gets somewhat overgrown and swampy in places. It is 6.6 miles to Bourne Pond and 8 miles to the west side of Stratton Pond. Long loops of 16 or 19 miles can be made by returning via the Branch Pond Trail or the LT/AT past Prospect Rock and down Old Rootville Road and East Manchester Road.

NEARBY A few miles north, you can make a challenging 3-mile round trip to **Prospect Rock** via Old Rootville Road, a rocky service road. The lower half is particularly steep, but the grade eases some near the top and the view across the deep valley below from the open ledge near the junction with the LT/AT is terrific. Parking is very limited, and the road is open to ORVs.

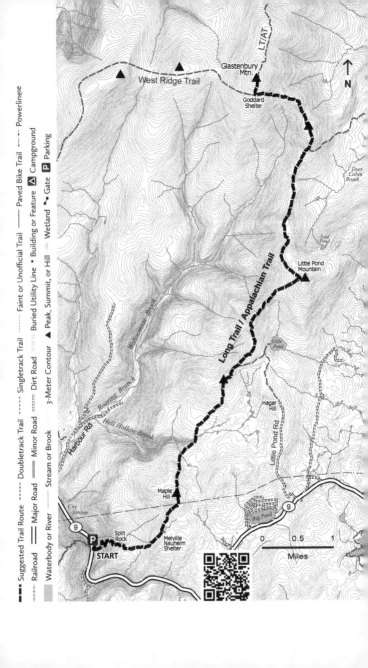

Suggested Trail Route   ----- Doubletrack Trail   ---- Singletrack Trail   .... Faint or Unofficial Trail   ——— Paved Bike Trail   +—+ Powerlinee

+++ Railroad   ——— Major Road   :::::: Minor Road   ······· Dirt Road   ⊕⊞⊟ Buried Utility Line   • Building or Feature   Δ Campground

——— Stream or Brook   ——— Waterbody or River   ——— 3-Meter Contour   ▲ Peak, Summit, or Hill   Wetland   • Gate   🅿 Parking

LT/AT

Glastenbury Mtn.

West Ridge Trail

Goddard Shelter

Deer Cabin Brook

Lost Pond

Little Pond Mountain

Long Trail / Appalachian Trail

Willowdale Brook

Roaring Branch

Little Pond

Hagar Hill

Harbour Rd

Hell Hollow Brook

Little Pond Rd

Maple Hill

City Stream

Big Pond

9

Split Rock

Melville Nauheim Shelter

9

🅿

START

N

0   0.5   1

Miles

DISTANCE 19.1 Miles **TOWN** Glastenbury

DIFFICULTY RATING Moderate/Challenging **TRAIL STYLE** Out-and-Back

TRAIL TYPE Singletrack **TOTAL ASCENT** 4,406 Feet

Despite its proximity to Bennington to the southwest, remote Glastenbury Mountain caps one of the largest areas of contiguous wilderness in the northeast. The 3,737-foot wooded summit features an observation deck on a former fire tower. Notable features along this section of the Long Trail/Appalachian Trail (LT/AT) include a scenic suspension bridge, glacial erratic boulders, two shelters, and scenic vistas. Though it is now cloaked in mature forest, most of the mountain and surrounding area was completely clearcut just a century ago. Several state-uncommon birds have since been documented here, and black bears are common.

DIRECTIONS From Bennington, take Rte. 9 east for 5 miles to the paved parking lot on the left. There is space for ~20–25 vehicles. Limited overflow parking could be available in the old gravel turnout on the other side of Rte. 9.

GPS: "LT/AT Trailhead, Woodford, VT"

TRAIL From the trailhead follow the gravel path east for a few hundred feet, then turn left to cross the suspension bridge over City Stream. Bear left and follow the white-blazed LT/AT west down the north bank of the stream. In a few hundred feet, turn sharply right and begin climbing steeply up the hillside out of the stream valley.

At 0.5 miles the trail rounds a ridge and there is a limited view northwest. Just above, pass through a short, narrow cleft between the two bisected halves of a large broken boulder called Split Rock. Then continue climbing, at a gentler grade now, for 0.8 miles nearly due east. After crossing several old woods roads, you'll arrive at a junction where a side trail leads 250 feet east to Melville Nauheim Shelter.

From the shelter junction, climb north at a moderate grade for 0.4 miles to a wide powerline swath with views east and west. Entering Glastenbury Wilderness on the other side of the powerline, continue north into the woods at an easy grade. In 0.1 mile, cross over the wooded top of 2,677-ft. Maple Hill. Descend gently north for nearly a mile to a crossing of upper Hell Hollow Brook, then climb at a gentle grade for another mile to a forested peak along the ridge. After passing a lookout with a view to the southeast, descend slightly for 0.2 miles to a junction where a relatively wide but somewhat soggy, blue-blazed side trail (Little Pond Link) leads east for 0.75 miles over and then down to the brushy shore of Little Pond.

Continue north on the LT/AT for 0.9 miles to a wooded peak, pass a ledge with a limited east-facing vista, then roll along the ridge another 0.9 miles, rising through scraggly old trees to yet another wooded peak (Little Pond Mountain). You are now ~6 miles north of Rte. 9. Keep rolling along the ridge for about 2 miles to a junction just past the Glastenbury Wilderness boundary line, passing several more lookouts and crossing a few more old woods roads along the way. Climb steadily for 1.3 miles, with a few level stretches and short dips punctuating the ascent, bearing north and then west up into spruce-fir forest and on to Goddard Shelter. There are several short but very steep rises just before the shelter.

Turn right at the shelter and climb due north for 0.3 miles to the wooded summit of Glastenbury Mountain, where the former fire tower had been converted to an observation deck with a 360-degree view; the tower was closed for safety reasons in 2022. From there, return back to the trailhead the way you came.

Optional Alternate Route You can turn the Glastenbury trek into a long, adventurous circuit loop by descending from the summit to the shelter then taking a right on the West Ridge Trail. Follow this trail, initially west and then south, for 7.4 miles to Bald Mountain and then take a left to descend the east side of Bald Mountain Trail to Old Harbour Road. Note that this option does require braving a dangerous, mile-long stretch of busy Rte. 9 at the end, where you're disconcertingly up against a metal guardrail with no road shoulder as traffic whizzes by.

NEARBY From the trailhead on the south side of Rte. 9, it is 3.3 miles round-trip up and back on the LT/AT to the top of 2,323-ft. **Harmon Hill**. The meadowy, savannah-like summit area features a nice westerly view out across Bennington and the Taconic Range, but the first half mile or so is very steep and technical, climbing a rugged stretch of rock stairs called The Thousand Steps. The full LT/AT section between Woodford and Rte. 2 in North Adams, MA is about 17 miles; though there is significant elevation change, with multiple named and unnamed peaks along the way, overall it features many pleasantly runnable stretches and makes a nice long, point-to point trail run.

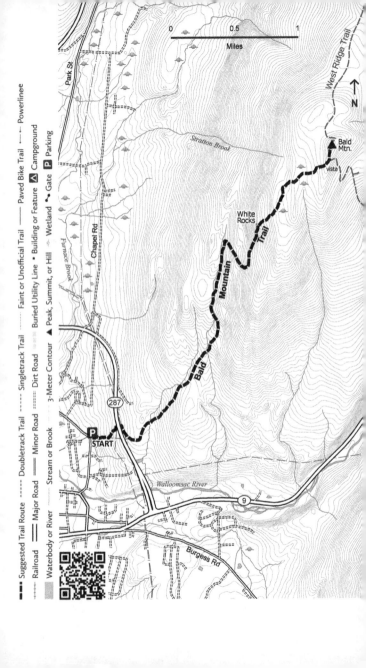

Suggested Trail Route ····· Doubletrack Trail ----- Singletrack Trail ---- Faint or Unofficial Trail ·····—·· Paved Bike Trail ·—·— Powerline
++++ Railroad ━━ Major Road ━━ Minor Road ┄┄┄┄ Dirt Road ┅┅┅ Buried Utility Line • Building or Feature Ⓐ Campground
━━ Waterbody or River ─── Stream or Brook ─── 3-Meter Contour ▲ Peak, Summit, or Hill ⬩ Wetland ● Gate Ⓟ Parking

0   0.5   1
Miles

West Ridge Trail

Stratton Brook

Bald Mtn.

vista

White Rocks

Mountain Trail

Chapel Rd

Furnace Brook

Park St

Bald

287

Ⓟ START

Walloomsac River

9

Burgess Rd

DISTANCE 7.8 Miles   **TOWN** Bennington and Woodford
DIFFICULTY RATING Moderate   **TRAIL STYLE** Out-and-Back
TRAIL TYPE Singletrack   **TOTAL ASCENT** 2,150 Feet

The western edge of the Green Mountains rises steeply and dramatically above a long stretch of north–south running Vermont Valley. Northeast of Bennington, 2,848-ft. Bald Mountain caps a prominent rise in the ridge, and a distinctive bare ledge called White Rocks stands out on its side, visible from many locations in the valley below. The full Bald Mountain Trail climbs up to the summit ridge and then goes down the other side to a separate trailhead in Woodford; this western portion is sometimes called the "White Rocks Trail" and the east side is sometimes called the "Bear Wallow Trail." The actual summit lies just north along the West Ridge Trail, which continues on for several miles to Glastenbury Mountain. Though there are several steep pitches, overall the grade is moderate. Footing is characteristically rocky and rooty throughout, except at the very top where the trailbed actually consists of a soft, fine white sand.

DIRECTIONS   From Bennington, take Rte. 9/Main St. east for 0.8 miles. Turn left on Branch Street and go 0.3 miles north. Turn right on North Branch Street, cross the brook and curve left, and go 0.4 miles north. At a bend to the left, take a right up an unmarked paved road just past a power line swath. The parking lot is on the right.

GPS: "White Rocks, North Branch Street, Bennington"

TRAIL   From the trailhead at the southeast corner of the lot, climb the wood-and-gravel crib steps up past the map kiosk into the open powerline swath. Zig-zag up through the shrubs for 0.2 miles then enter the woods on the north side. Look for blue blazes. In a few hundred feet, bear right on an old rocky woods road and climb for 0.1 mile up into a narrow chute formed by metal fences. Follow the chute to a spacious, graffiti-garnished underpass beneath the Rte. 279 bypass road and proceed through.

Exit the fence-lined chute on the other side of the tunnel, then turn right and climb 0.1 mile at a gentle grade up into an open powerline swath meadow above and east of the roadway. Follow the trail back into the woods on the far side where it enters Green Mountain National Forest.

At a moderate grade, climb 0.8 miles northeast up the slope along wide old woods roads through northern hardwood forest to a Forest Service sign, passing junctions and intersections with a warren of other, unmarked woods roads along the way. At the sign, cross into the protected Glastenbury Wilderness. The pathway narrows to more of a singletrack hiking trail in this area. Along a somewhat rugged stretch, the trail crosses several streams and bypasses a few wet areas. Some parts may be muddy here. In the middle of this section, the trail briefly rises along a ribbon of conspicuously bare, moss-lined bedrock ledge.

At 0.9 miles from the wilderness boundary, swing hard right and climb diagonally southeast up the slope at a steeper grade. In 0.3 miles, swing left and climb a short steep pitch while entering a zone of mixed spruce-fir and northern hardwood forest, then ascend 0.3 miles north. After passing a faint herd path down into a small rocky open area, you'll pass just below a treeless area of loose rocks above to the right. Just before reaching the open area, look for a small rock cairn along the trail. It marks a spur path on the left that leads a short distance over to a ledge at the upper part of the White Rocks slide; from here there is a wide-ranging view out over Vermont Valley, the Taconics, and the Hudson Valley to the west.

Continuing north from the White Rocks spur, cross the first open rocky patch, marked with a large rubble-pile cairn, then pass through several more. The footing is tricky over loose cobbles and sharp stones. After passing into spruce-fir forest, cross a wooded ridge, descend to several low, wet saddles, and then rise gently through increasingly stunted spruce and fir trees to a junction with West Ridge Trail, marked by a cairn with a trail sign. It is 0.8 miles from White Rocks to this junction.

The windswept summit ridge of Bald Mountain is notable for its thin layer of light, sandy soil, making the trail look like a moss-and-lichen-lined white ribbon through the dark green boreal forest trees. Follow the gentle curves of West Ridge Trail 0.1 mile north up the ridge to the true summit, marked by a low, broad cairn, where there is a view north towards Glastenbury Mountain. Return to the trailhead the way you came up.

> *Optional Extension* From Bald Mountain, the lightly traveled but scenic West Ridge Trail continues north along the rugged ridgecrest for another 7.4 miles to Goddard Shelter and a junction with the Long Trail/Appalachian Trail just below Glastenbury Mountain. Note to photographers: the moss-lined trail leading north down off the summit of Bald Mountain is particularly pretty.

NEARBY About a mile northwest of this trailhead, there is a very small trail network at **Maneely Park** in Bennington (the short trail loop at nearby **Willow Park** is paved).

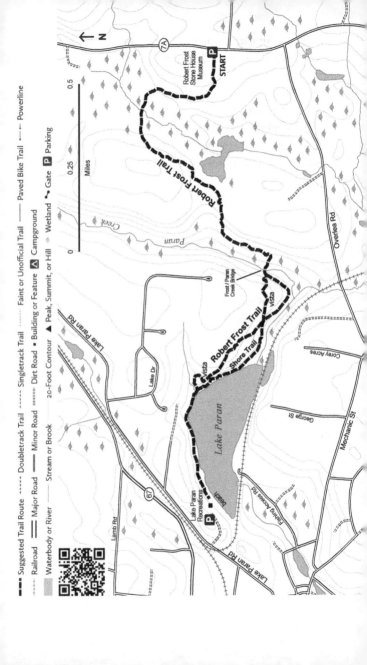

← N

Suggested Trail Route · · · · · Doubletrack Trail · · · · · Singletrack Trail · · · · · Faint or Unofficial Trail — · — Paved Bike Trail — · · — Powerline
+++++ Railroad ═══ Major Road ═══ Minor Road ═══ Dirt Road ▪ Building or Feature ▲ Campground
▬▬▬ Waterbody or River ─── Stream or Brook ─── 20-Foot Contour ▲ Peak, Summit, or Hill ◇ Wetland ⌐ Gate 🅿 Parking

0   0.25   0.5
Miles

Robert Frost Stone House Museum
🅿 START

Paran Creek

Robert Frost Trail

Frost / Paran Creek Bridge

vista

Robert Frost Trail

vista

Shore Trail

Lake Paran

Lake Paran Recreations
🅿

Lake Paran Rd

Lake Dr

Lamb Rd

67

Overlea Rd

Corey Acres

George St

Mechanic St

Fishing Access Rd

7A

DISTANCE 4.2 Miles   **TOWN** Shaftsbury and Bennington
DIFFICULTY RATING Easy/Moderate   **TRAIL STYLE** Out-and-Back
TRAIL TYPE Singletrack   **TOTAL ASCENT** 285 Feet

The Robert Frost Trail, which opened for use in 2011, runs roughly two miles east–west between the Robert Frost Stone House Museum in southern Shaftsbury and Lake Paran in North Bennington. Marked with blue paint blazes, the trail gently rolls up and down across low wooded hills of the valley floor, crossing Paran Creek, passing through several forest types, and skirting the edge of Lake Paran. There are several scenic vistas of the surrounding mountains beyond. At the eastern end of the trail is the property where Robert Frost lived from 1920 to 1928; in 1923 he wrote "Stopping by Woods on a Snowy Evening" there. If it's hot, you can start from the west side at the town park and take a swim at the beach afterwards (there is an admission fee to enter Paran Recreation's Lake Paran park). Bicycles are not permitted on the Robert Frost Trail.

DIRECTIONS   From Rte. 7 north of Bennington, take Rte. 7A north for 3.1 miles to the Robert Frost Stone House Museum entrance driveway on the left. The short dirt drive to the trailhead parking lot is immediately on the left. Please do not park in the museum parking lot.
GPS: "Robert Frost Trailhead (East) Shaftsbury"

TRAIL   From the trailhead sign at the west end of the parking lot, follow the wide, mown path 0.1 mile west across a small grassy field and enter the woods on the far side. Curve right and go 0.3 miles north through woods that include the scattered remnant trees of an old apple orchard and a stand of red pines planted by Robert Frost.

Descend slightly to cross a low, narrow, vegetated causeway across a wetland creek, then head southwest and skirt the northern edge of a wetland. Then pass along the right side of an open meadow. Dipping back into the woods, curve left and pass through the narrow Paran Creek valley among occasional stone ledges and outcrops. Cross a covered wooden bridge over Paran Creek (watch your heads, tall runners); at 1.1 miles, this marks the halfway point.

On the west side of the bridge, at a fork where a branch of the Shore Trail leads left (the branches rejoin in about half a mile), stay straight and climb a short steep hill to a small field with an expansive view of the surrounding landscape. Continuing west, dip down to a low point with junctions where the first Shore Trail branch rejoins and the second leads left towards the lake (the second set of branches rejoin in 0.6 miles). Bear right again and climb a low, grassy hill where there is a viewpoint overlooking the west side of the lake. After a short, steep descent you'll come to another fork where the second Shore Trail branch rejoins. Go straight and cross a long stretch of wide boardwalks over a marshy fringe right along the north side of the lake, then stay straight on a wide, gently undulating grassy stretch through the woods.

The path ends at the edge of the trees where the accessible concrete sidewalk leading to the beach from the bathhouse above makes a hairpin turn. To return, go back the way you came but for variety make sure to take the alternate paths to the ones you took before, the Shore Trail branches that trace the edges of Lake Paran and Paran Creek, respectively. These trails not only feature nice waterside views but also pass through pretty white birch stands and make use of well-built wooden steps to negotiate sensitive, easily eroded slopes.

NEARBY The **Mile-Around Woods** site (see Site 16) is located about a mile to the southwest.

DISTANCE 2.7 Miles   **TOWN** Bennington
DIFFICULTY RATING Easy   **TRAIL STYLE** Loop
TRAIL TYPE Doubletrack/Singletrack   **TOTAL ASCENT** 225 Feet

The Mile-Around Woods features a network of mostly gentle trails centered around a wide, flowy carriage trail loop through a mix of old forests and working agricultural fields. The trails are neither marked nor signed, but they are easy to follow. This suggested route roughly traces the outer perimeter of the site's trail network, though other smaller loops can easily be added on or repeated throughout. The Mile-Around Woods property is especially notable for its showy displays of ephemeral wildflowers in the spring. Dogs must be leashed in the central woods portion as well as on roads leading to it, and bicycles are not permitted on the Mile-Around Woods trails.

DIRECTIONS   From Rte. 7 in Bennington, take Rte. 67A north for 2.7 miles to the village of North Bennington. Turn left on West Street/ McCullough Road and go 0.4 miles west to parking along the left side of the road. There is also parking just to the east at the Park-McCullough House lot.

GPS: "Mile-Around Woods, Woods Lane"

TRAIL   At the trailhead, go around the gate and follow the wide, fence-lined dirt road (Woods Lane) south across the open field, curving slightly left, for 0.1 mile to a junction. Take a right and rise gently along a maple-tree-lined dirt road for 0.15 miles to a junction by a bench in the woods just past an open metal gate.

Go straight and then immediately bear left at a fork in the road. The wide dirt trail rolls through the woods along the east side of a hill for 0.5 miles, passing boulders and views along the way. At a junction where a

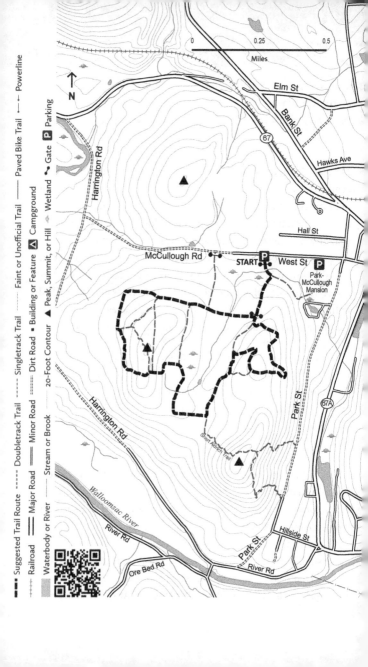

Suggested Trail Route · · · · Doubletrack Trail - - - - Faint or Unofficial Trail —— Paved Bike Trail ⊢—⊣ Powerline
⊢⊢⊢⊢ Railroad · · · · · Singletrack Trail :::::::::: Dirt Road —— Minor Road —— Major Road ⚫ Building or Feature ▲ Campground
—— Waterbody or River —— Stream or Brook —— 20-Foot Contour ▲ Peak, Summit, or Hill ⋋ Wetland ⬥ Gate 🅿 Parking

0   0.25   0.5
Miles

N

Elm St

Bank St

67

Hawks Ave

Harrington Rd

Hall St

McCullough Rd

START 🅿 West St 🅿

Park-
McCullough
Mansion

Harrington Rd

Park St

67A

Short Aldrich Trail

Walloomsac River

River Rd

Hillside St

Park St

River Rd

Ore Bed Rd

narrower hiking trail leads left, bear right and follow the trail 0.2 miles down some curves to a junction. Take a left and go 0.1 mile south up to a junction. Go right and follow the singletrack trail a few hundred feet south down through the woods to a bench at the edge of a field.

Follow the trail along the upper, east side of the field 0.15 miles to a junction where the Short Aldrich Trail continues south. Take a right and follow the mowed trail west for 0.15 miles across the field. Follow a curve to the right and go north for 0.2 miles to a junction. Go left and follow the path for 0.15 miles west as it traces the southern edge of a field. At a junction, go straight into the woods.

Follow the trail for 0.25 miles west and north down through the woods to a junction. Bear left and emerge at the eastern edge of a field. Turn right and follow the upper edge of the field for 0.25 miles. Curve right and follow the trail steeply up the hill to a junction. Stay straight and follow the trail east across the open field to a junction with a trail on the right. Stay straight and keep going east, passing a junction with a dirt road on the left and in a few hundred feet and then descending to a junction with a dirt road leading south to a barn on the right. Stay straight, cross a low area, and in 0.15 miles reach a junction. Take a left and return to the trailhead the way you came in.

Optional Extensions Several connecting trails run north–south through the center of the property and can be used to make short loops, mostly out in open fields. On the south side of the site, the Short Aldrich Trail leads 0.5 miles across and then down the hillside to Park Street.

NEARBY The **Lake Paran** site is located about a mile to the northeast. On the east side of Paran Creek below Mile-Around Woods, a short, somewhat hard-to-find trail traces the hillside west of **Bennington College** above the creek. Just across the state line in New York, combine the Battle Loop and Valley View Trails at **Bennington Battlefield State Historic Site** in Hoosick for a hilly, 3-mile figure-8 route with excellent views.

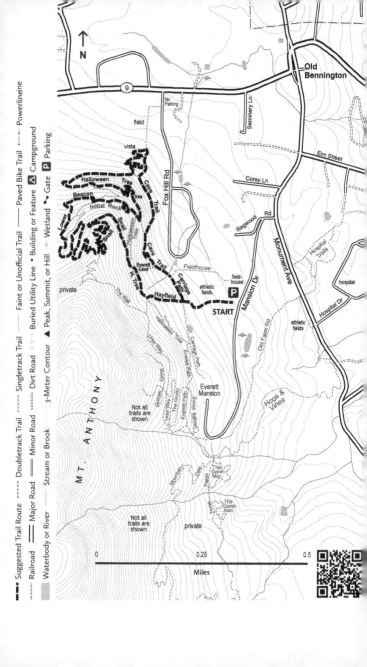

Legend:

- ▮ Suggested Trail Route
- ---- Doubletrack Trail
- ----- Singletrack Trail
- ---- Faint or Unofficial Trail
- — Paved Bike Trail
- +-+ Powerlinene
- +++ Railroad
- ━━ Major Road
- ═══ Minor Road
- ┉┉┉ Dirt Road
- ┄┄┄ Buried Utility Line
- ▪ Building or Feature
- ▲ Campground
- — Stream or Brook
- ▒ Waterbody or River
- 〰 3-Meter Contour
- ▲ Peak, Summit, or Hill
- ⬗ Wetland
- ⌐ Gate
- ℗ Parking

N ↑

Old Bennington

(9)

No Parking

field

vista

Halloween Tree

Beacon

Initial Rock

Lower

Small Small

Halloween Tree

Cave Tree

Cave Trail

Cave Trail

Everett Cave

H Tree

Hayfield

The Wall

private

Seminary Ln

Elm Street

Corey Ln

Regwood Rd

Monument Ave

Hospital Trails

hospital

Hospital Dr

athletic fields

Fox Hill Rd

Fieldhouse

field-house

athletic fields

Carriage Path

START

℗

Mansion Dr

Old Farm Rd

Halloween Trail

Carriage Path

Everett Path

Everett Mansion

Hops & Vines

Long Way

Genies

Grotto

Unsa Way

The Grotto

Everett Path

Everett Bypass

M T.   A N T H O N Y

Not all trails are shown

Mountain

Corey Fields

The Green Man

The Green Man

Not all trails are shown

private

0   0.25   0.5

Miles

DISTANCE 3.9 Miles   **TOWN** Bennington
DIFFICULTY RATING Moderate   **TRAIL STYLE** Loop
TRAIL TYPE Singletrack   **TOTAL ASCENT** 690 Feet

As a relative monadnock peak within the greater Taconic Mountain Range, 2,343-ft. Mount Anthony towers alone over the southwest side of the city of Bennington. The well-marked, well-maintained, and well-loved Bennington Area Trail System (BATS) laces the lower north-eastern slopes of the mountain, providing magnificent recreational opportunities for the local community and visitors alike. Over eight miles of trails pass through rich forests and scenic meadows, and visit interesting geologic and historic features throughout. Difficulties range from easy to very challenging, with colored BATS trail markers serving as blazes. BATS trails are located on private property and are generously open for public use. The closure of Southern Vermont College (SVC) and other recent changes in land ownership mean that the specific public access points to some of the lower trails and mown paths by the old SVC campus may shift in the future.

DIRECTIONS From Bennington, take Rte. 9/West Road west for 1 mile. Turn left on Monument Avenue and go south for 0.6 miles. Turn right on Regwood Road. In 250 feet, turn left onto Mansion Drive and go 0.4 miles up to the parking lot by the field house on the right, following signs for "Mt. Anthony Trails (BATS)." At the time of writing, parking is allowed here.

GPS: "Bennington Area Trail System, Mansion Drive"

TRAIL From the fieldhouse parking area, head up the grassy slope to the west on an unnamed path and climb past playing fields on the right. At a junction, bear right and follow Carriage Path north along the edge of the woods above the fields. At a junction with Fieldhouse trail on the right, go straight and continue northwest on the relatively easy Cave Trail. It soon passes a steep spur path on the left leading to a cool cavern in the rock ledge called Everett Cave (you can go into it, so bring a headlamp).

Continue north on Cave Trail, passing several connector paths leading left up the slope. After gently rolling along the slope for a bit, descend to a junction just above an open field. Take a sharp left and follow the red-blazed Halloween Tree Trail, which switchbacks up the slope at gentle grades for 0.6 miles, passing several junctions with linking trails on the left. At a signed junction, bear left to stay on Halloween Tree Trail, which playfully and gently winds and rolls around the hillside for 0.3 miles to the actual Halloween Tree, a huge, ultra-scraggly old maple trunk with decorations.

From the tree, go 0.1 mile south across the slope to a junction with MAPS Connector Trail. Turn sharply right to stay on Halloween Tree and climb 0.1 mile to a junction. Turn right and follow Initial Rock Trail 0.2 miles west across the slope to an intersection, passing the namesake rock about halfway along.

Go right on the green-blazed Lower Beacon and follow it 0.2 miles west and south up to a junction with a connector trail going left/east. Bear right to stay on Lower Beacon again and follow it 0.1 mile up to an upper junction with Initial Rock Trail. Take a right to stay on Lower Beacon yet again and follow it 0.6 miles up multiple switchbacks (and passing a Crossover Trail on the left leading over to Snail Trail) to a junction near the crest of the mountain's north ridge. You'll see the actual beacon here. Lower Beacon Trail actually continues climbing a little higher up the ridge to the right/south but it's also a little more technical.

Take a left and begin descending on Snail Trail. After 0.6 miles of steadily dropping down switchbacks you'll arrive at a junction with red-blazed Halloween Tree Trail. Follow Halloween Tree Trail 0.15 mile southeast to an intersection. Turn left and follow Hayfield/Ursa Way down a mown path through an open field. The grade is moderately steep here. At an intersection with Carriage Path, go straight down the open hillside to return to the trailhead.

Optional Extensions This route is just a sampling of the BATS trail network. Enjoyable extension options are plentiful here. For example, Everett Path/Everett Ballcourt Trails pass some interesting old structures in the woods above Everett Mansion. Some other notable trails to explore include Hops and Vines, Ursa Way, Grimes' Grind, The Grotto, The Green Man, Running Bear, Jacob's Ladder, and Mountain Dew.

NEARBY Just to the east, immediately across Monument Avenue from the lower end of the BATS network's Hops and Vines trail, there are several trail loops called **Hospital Trails** and **Hospital Loops** in the woods northwest of Southwestern Vermont Medical Center (SVMC); these are accessible from a small parking pull-off along Monument Avenue. About a mile or so to the east, the **Greenberg Conservation Reserve** on the east side of Rte. 7 supports a small network of short trails through fields and woods bordering a wetland. Close by, the **Greenburg Headwaters Park** has two miles of gentle, unmarked trails amid forest and wetlands; the primary parking and trailhead is at the end of Belvidere Street.

A few miles southwest, the **Taconic Crest Trail** stretches north–south for 37 miles along the top of the Taconic Mountains, with the northern part briefly swinging into the southwestern corner of Vermont. A strenuous 4.7-mile climb up the steep trail from the parking area at its northern terminus along New York Rte. 346 will bring you to an interesting geologic fissure called the **Snow Hole** (just west of the New York/Vermont state line).

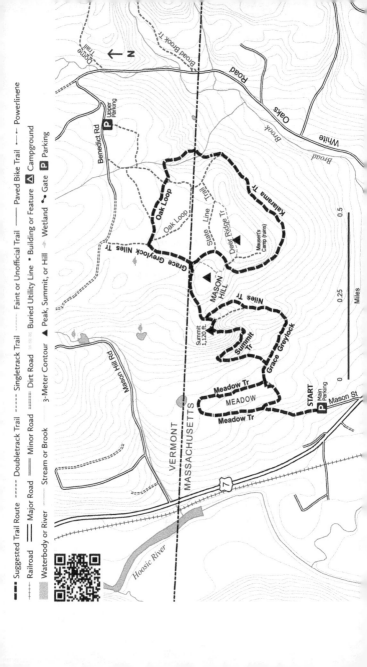

18 Mountain Meadow Preserve

DISTANCE 3.7 Miles **TOWN** Pownal, VT and Williamstown, MA
DIFFICULTY RATING Moderate **TRAIL STYLE** Figure-8 Loop
TRAIL TYPE Singletrack/Doubletrack **TOTAL ASCENT** 530 Feet

Straddling the Vermont/Massachusetts state line, The Trustees'
Mountain Meadow Preserve hosts a network of marked trails that
are easily accessible from entry points in either state. The mostly
south-sloping landscape primarily consists of rolling hills, steep
ridges, pocket wetlands, and sprawling meadows, the latter of which
fill with wildflowers in spring and summer. The lower and upper parts
offer considerably easier travel, while the steep slopes between the
two require more effort to tackle. This suggested route around the
perimeter of the property offers a representative sampling of the terrain. Be aware that in the upper part of the property you will encounter
numerous unofficial and/or unmapped trails, some even marked with
wooden signs (e.g., Deer Ridge Trail, Tom's Trail, Hillside Trail,
Roundabout, etc.); some of these may be a bit rougher but they can
be fun, especially as backcountry ski trails in winter.

DIRECTIONS From Rte. 7 in Williamstown, MA, about 0.7 miles
south of the VT/MA state line, take Mason Street north to a parking
lot at the end. There is also a sizable parking area off of Benedict
Road (dirt) in Pownal, VT.

GPS: "Mountain Meadow Preserve, Mason Street"

TRAIL From the trailhead, take the Niles Trail 0.2 miles north to
a junction. Turn right and stay on Niles as you curve left around an
open meadow and gently climb 0.1 mile to an overlook.

From the overlook, descend slightly to a junction with Meadow
Trail, then go right to stay on Niles Trail, entering the woods and

immediately crossing a small bridge. Stay right on Niles at three successive marked junctions as you climb, sometimes steeply, up the slope for 0.7 miles. Then, at a junction just south of the state line, stay straight on Mausert's Camp Trail (the Niles Trail goes left). In 0.1 mile, after passing a rough Skier's Hill Trail leading uphill to the right, bear right at a junction with State & Town Line Trail and go another 0.1 mile to a junction.

Optional Extension A short spur road leads left about 0.1 mile up to Mausert's Camp just below the top of 1,125-ft. Mason Hill.

At the junction, take Kalarama Trail, initially down past another junction with Skier's Hill Trail and then curving left around the side of Mason Hill. Multiple marked and unmarked woods roads and trails cross Kalarama; keep following the yellow blazes and signs. In 0.6 miles, bear right to stay on Kalarama where State Line Trail leads left. Drop 0.1 mile down the hill and cross a stream, then climb 0.3 miles up to a junction. Go right and then immediately left at another junction.

Go 0.2 miles west on the mostly flat Oak Loop trail to a junction, then go straight a few hundred feet to another junction. Turn left and go south on Greylock Niles Trail for 0.15 miles to a junction just past the VT/MA state line. Turn right on Niles and go 0.2 miles to a junction. Bear right/straight on Summit Trail and climb a short distance to a junction. Turn right and cross over the top of a 1,120-ft. wooded peak with no views, then drop steeply down the hillside for 0.4 miles on a long zig-zag switchback.

At the bottom, go right on Niles again, then turn right on Meadow back out in the open. Loop 0.5 miles around the meadow for a final, pleasant jog through open-field scenery. Return to the trailhead on the Niles Trail.

NEARBY From a trailhead along White Oaks Road right at the VT/MA state line you can make a 5-mile semi-loop run of **The Dome**, a southern Green Mountains peak in Pownal. From the trailhead parking area, head first at a gentle grade up the scenic Broad Brook Trail, then after about a mile swing left and climb very steeply up the rugged Agawon Trail (not recommended for descending) to the Dome Trail on the ridge. Turn right and ascend more gradually north to the summit. Most of the route is through deciduous forest but at 2,743 feet the very top passes through a dark canopy of spruce and fir trees with lush green moss underneath. There is a limited view south from white-colored rock ledges. Descend via the Dome Trail and then return to the trailhead on White Oaks Road (dirt). This overall moderately challenging route is quite rocky in places and tends to be very muddy in spring. In general, Williamstown, MA is loaded with other great trail-running opportunities, including close-by **Pine Cobble** and **Hopkins Memorial Forest**, both just south of the state line (for full site profiles, see *Trail Running Western Massachusetts*).

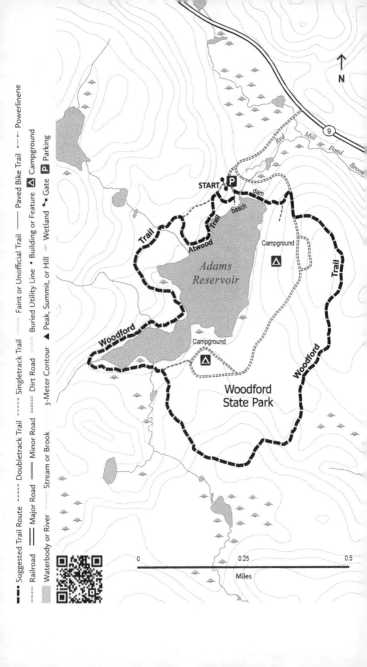

Suggested Trail Route ••• Doubletrack Trail ---- Singletrack Trail ..... Faint or Unofficial Trail —— Paved Bike Trail ⊢—⊣ Powerline/ine

++++ Railroad ══ Major Road ▒▒▒ Minor Road ∷∷∷ Dirt Road ••• Buried Utility Line • Building or Feature ▲ Campground

━━ Waterbody or River —— Stream or Brook — 3-Meter Contour ▲ Peak, Summit, or Hill ⚶ Wetland ⚬ Gate **P** Parking

N

START **P**

dam

beach

Atwood Trail

Campground

Adams Reservoir

Trail

Woodford

Campground

Woodford State Park

Woodford

Trail

9

Red Mill Pond Brook

0   0.25   0.5

Miles

DISTANCE 2.4 Miles   **TOWN** Woodford
DIFFICULTY RATING Easy/Moderate   **TRAIL STYLE** Loop
TRAIL TYPE Singletrack   **TOTAL ASCENT** 210 Feet

While most suggested routes in this guide are at least 3 miles long, it's worth making an exception for Woodford State Park. The Woodford Trail that loops around the lake here is absolutely splendid either for a short run or multiple loops. Marked with blue rectangular blazes and signed at all junctions, the trail is easy to follow and features multiple lakeside vistas as well as beautiful, fern-lined forest settings. The grade is mostly gentle and the footing is generally good, though there are the usual rocks and roots of all Vermont trails through-out. Located at a relatively high elevation (2,400 feet) on the plateau between Bennington and Wilmington, the 400-acre park is nearly surrounded by the Green Mountain National Forest, and a portion of the trail passes through the George D. Aiken Wilderness Area. With its short length and easy navigability, this makes a good site for first-time trail runners. As a bonus, you can also cool off with a swim at the beach afterwards in summer.

DIRECTIONS   From Wilmington, take Rte. 9 west for 10 miles to the park entrance on the left. Park in the Day-Use lot just past the entrance station. From Bennington, take Rte. 9 east for 11 miles to the park entrance on the right. There is an entrance fee, and in the winter the park access road is closed at a gate just south of Rte. 9.

GPS: "Woodford State Park"

TRAIL   From the dirt parking lot, continue down towards the water. The main trailhead is on the right, marked "Reservoir Loop Trail" (and labeled "Reservoir Trail" on some maps). Follow the trail west up the hill into the woods at a gentle grade, curving slightly to the right. At a junction where a dirt road path leads back down to the parking lot, go left on the Woodford Trail. In a few hundred feet, go left at a fork where the main trail leads straight ahead. This side trail is called the Atwood Trail.

Drop 0.1 mile down through the woods to Adams Reservoir and follow the trail for 0.15 miles along the edge of the pond, crossing occasional boardwalks and passing several scenic vistas out over the water. Curve right and climb gradually for 0.1 mile back up to a junction with the main trail. Go left and follow the trail 0.6 miles around the southwest side of the pond, rising and falling slightly along the way. At a wooden bridge over an inlet stream, curve left and go 0.1 mile east to a junction where a side trail leads several hundred feet east to the park campground.

Take a right and climb uphill at an easy grade, soon passing a sign marking the boundary of the George D. Aiken Wilderness Area. The trail soon levels out. Gradually curve left above the edge of a wetland, cross back into the state park, and go north through the woods. The trail undulates slightly across the forested landscape, crossing a few wet areas and passing a few ledges and boulders, until it reaches the campground road. It is 1.2 miles from the junction by the pond to the park road.

Turn right and follow the paved road north for a few hundred feet. At a brown "Trail" sign with an arrow, take a left back into the woods. Very soon afterwards, at a fork marked with a "Reservoir Loop Trail" sign, go right and follow the path down the hill to the edge of the pond. Head west and cross the grassy dam and a small bridge back to the trailhead by the beach.

NEARBY A few miles west, **Prospect Mountain Ski Area** in Woodford features a network of winter-use trails for cross-country and back-country skiing as well as snowshoeing and snowshoe running. The trails aren't specifically maintained for summer use. To the northwest, it's a relatively easy 4-mile round-trip trek on a mix of old road and hiking trails up and over 2,759-ft. Hagar Hill to isolated **Little Pond**; from there, an extra half-mile link trail leads west to a junction with the Long Trail/Appalachian Trail.

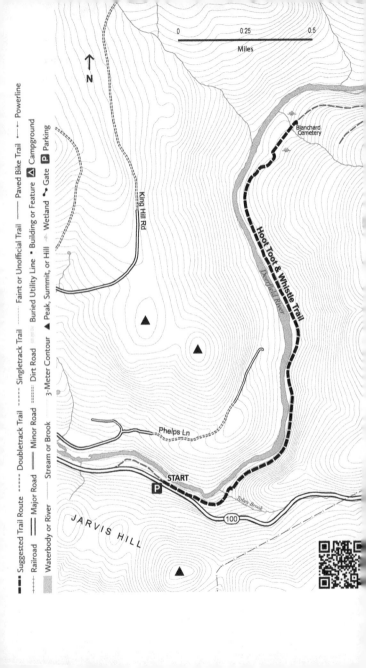

DISTANCE 3.7 Miles   **TOWN** Readsboro

DIFFICULTY RATING Easy   **TRAIL STYLE** Out-and-Back

TRAIL TYPE Singletrack   **TOTAL ASCENT** 220 Feet

The Hoot Toot & Whistle Trail is an old railroad bed, abandoned in 1937, that runs along the east side of the Deerfield River and Harriman Reservoir. The nickname comes from the old Hoosac Tunnel and Wilmington Railroad name, which was abbreviated to HT&W. Only certain sections are currently open as trails. This part coincides with the Catamount Trail ski corridor and is marked as such (blue diamond blazes with a black cat-paw print and "Catamount X-C Ski Trail" labels). It is generally flat and level, though the footing varies, with occasional rocky and wet areas along the way. Be aware that this section of river is dam-controlled and water levels are subject to change at any time.

DIRECTIONS   From Readsboro, take Rte. 100 north for 0.2 miles to the dirt parking lot on the hillside to the right.

GPS: "7748 Vermont Rte. 100 Readsboro"

TRAIL   From the parking lot, carefully cross Rte. 100 and find the trail in the brush at the edge of the woods on the other side (look for the blue Catamount Trail markers). Go right and follow the trail a few hundred feet east, immediately parallel to the road. Veer left at a boulder and follow the trail down an old road grade with rock ledges on the right to a ferny wooded terrace above the east side of the river. Cross a few eroded streamlets and wet areas, then cross a sturdy wooden pedestrian bridge over a sizable tributary creek at about 0.25 miles.

On the other side of the bridge, continue northeast along the terrace for a short distance, then swing sharply right for a quick climb up to a rock cut for the old rail grade. Turn left and continue heading northeast on the trail; this rock-wall flanked section is often somewhat muddy. Back out in more open forest, the trail soon begins to curve slightly left and trends northward. The Deerfield River periodically comes into view through the trees down below to the left.

At about 1 mile, the trail curves slightly northwest then continues straight ahead for a lengthy stretch. At around 1.5 miles, after a notable curve to the right, the trail veers to the right off the old rail grade to avoid a washed-out section. This is the trickiest footing of the route, though it isn't difficult. Cross a small stream on some rocks, then rejoin the rail bed heading northeast.

At 1.85 miles you will arrive at Blanchard Cemetery on the right, marked with a sign. To return to the trailhead, go back the same way you came in.

Optional Extension From the cemetery, the trail continues north for another half mile or so up to the Harriman Reservoir dam, though the last part that switchbacks up through a powerline to the parking area can be overgrown and somewhat hard to follow in summer. The part just north of the cemetery is quite narrow and dramatic as it hugs the steep, ledgy hillside above the river.

NEARBY At the northern end of Harriman Reservoir in Wilmington, a northern section of the **Hoot Toot & Whistle Trail** traces the south bank of the North Branch Deerfield River for 2 miles, linking the Reardon's Crossing pedestrian bridge in the village with the boat launch and swimming area at the end of Fairview Avenue; the 4-mile round trip is mostly flat and easy, though considerably rocky and rooty west of the crushed-gravel section near the water treatment plant. A rolling, 7-mile section of the **Catamount Trail** runs north–south along the west side of Harriman Reservoir between Woods Road at the north end and the dam at the south end (Harriman Station); access from the northern end. Just south across the state line in Massachusetts, there is a terrific (but notably challenging) 10-mile lollipop loop trail route at **Monroe State Forest**.

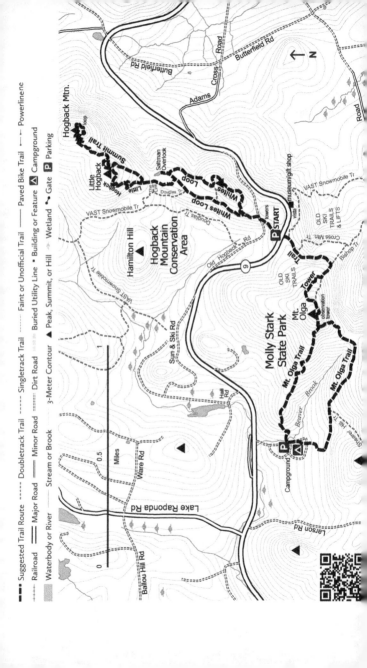

Legend:
- ■■■ Suggested Trail Route
- ---- Doubletrack Trail
- ········ Singletrack Trail
- ---- Faint or Unofficial Trail
- —— Paved Bike Trail
- — Powerline
- +++ Railroad
- === Major Road
- :::::: Minor Road
- ===== Dirt Road
- ---- Buried Utility Line
- ▪ Building or Feature
- ▲ Campground
- —— Waterbody or River
- —— Stream or Brook
- —— 3-Meter Contour
- ▲ Peak, Summit, or Hill
- ⟜ Wetland
- ● Gate
- P Parking

Hogback Mtn.
Loop
Summit Trail
Little Hogback
Little Hogback
Saltman Overlook
Douglas Tr
Whites Loop
Whites Loop
museum/gift shop
VAST Snowmobile Tr
Towers
START
P
OLD SKI TRAILS & LIFTS
Cross Mtn. Tr
Bishop Tr
VAST Snowmobile Tr
Hamilton Hill
Hogback Mountain Conservation Area
Douglas Tr
Old Hogback Rd
9
OLD SKI TRAILS
Tower Trail
Mt. Olga
conservation tower
Molly Stark State Park
VAST Snowmobile Tr
Sun & Ski Rd
Mt. Olga Trail
Beaver Brook
Mt. Olga Trail
Hall Rd
Shearer Hill Tr
Campground
P
A
Larson Rd
Lake Raponda Rd
Ware Rd
Ballou Hill Rd
Butterfield Rd
Adams Cross Road
Butterfield Rd
Road
← N

0   0.5   1
Miles

DISTANCE 6 Miles   **TOWN** Marlboro

DIFFICULTY RATING Moderate   **TRAIL STYLE** Figure-8 Loop

TRAIL TYPE Singletrack   **TOTAL ASCENT** 990 Feet

Early European settlers in New England used the term "hogback" to
describe a cluster of connected hills or peaks; in this case, the cluster includes 2,409-ft. Hogback Mountain, 2,354-ft. Little Hogback
Mountain, and 2,418-ft. Mount Olga as well as several unnamed hills
along the ridge in between. The Hogback Mountain Conservation
Area, which is bisected by Rte. 9, protects much of it through the
efforts of Hogback Mountain Conservation Association (HMCA),
while Molly Stark State Park includes the summit of Mount Olga
and its western slopes. The landscape is rolling hills, with a mix of
trail surface types. Rocks and roots are plentiful. In the middle is the
current museum/gift shop and associated infrastructure. South of Rte.
9, the overgrown remains of the former Hogback Ski Area trails lace
the eastern slopes of Mount Olga, and many of the old buildings and
lift structures are still there. This suggested route, consisting of two
distinct halves, uses many of the interconnected trails in the network
at the site and visits a variety of natural features.

DIRECTIONS   From I-91 in Brattleboro, take Rte. 9 west for 13.5 miles
to the top of the pass. The large parking lot is on the right.

GPS: "Hogback and Mount Olga Trailhead Parking"

TRAIL   *Loop 1: Hogback Mountain (3 miles)*   From the trailhead at
the back of the parking lot, start northeast up the white-blazed trail
past the boulders and into the woods. In 0.1 mile, go right on Old
Hogback Road, then immediately take a left into the woods at a sign
on the other side. Go 0.1 mile north to a junction, then take a right.

Follow the east side of White's Loop trail 0.3 miles up and over a hill to a junction with MES Cutoff trail. The trail surface here is quite rooty, and notably tends to hold the previous fall's leaves until well into the start of summer when other nearby trails are leaf-free. Take a right to continue following White's Trail north for about 0.25 miles along the east side of the ridge. After a curve to the west, go right at a junction to follow a short spur down to Saltman Overlook above the edge of a vernal pool.

Return to the junction from the pool, then continue straight. Take a right and go 0.1 mile north on Hogback Summit Trail to a junction with Link Trail on the left, then go straight a few hundred feet to a fork where the Little Hogback Trail goes left. Take a right and climb 0.2 miles up to an upper fork. Bear right and follow the white-blazed Hogback Summit Trail 0.3 miles down to a saddle and then up to a junction just past some ledges on Hogback Mountain.

Go left to start following the red-blazed, 0.15-mile loop around the summit. Back at the fork, descend south on Summit Trail back to the fork with Little Hogback Trail. Bear right to take the Little Hogback Trail branch this time; it switchbacks 0.4 miles south across and down Little Hogback Mountain to the lower fork. Then go straight and follow the Summit Trail 0.2 miles south back across the saddle, passing the junction with the Link Trail on the right along the way.

Take a right to follow the west side of White's Loop trail south for 0.4 miles across the west slope of the hill, passing junctions with Douglas Trail on the right and MES Cutoff on the left. Go straight at the junction and return to the trailhead the way you came in.

Optional Extensions Hogback Mountain Conservation Area includes a few more trails. From the Douglas Trail on the west side of Hogback Mountain (which is just below the suggested route and can be linked to from it), a VAST snowmobile route called the Raponda Ridge Trail leads 1.2 miles west over to the hillside above Lake Raponda, but does not go down to the lake. The Douglas Trail itself is not as well maintained as the rest of this network and can be challenging to follow.

Loop 2: Mount Olga (3 miles)   Carefully cross busy Rte. 9 and find the start of Tower Trail on the right/west side of a building. Take the wide Tower Trail southwest up the hill for 0.7 miles to the fire tower at the top. Along the way, the trail passes multiple junctions with Rim Run, Cross-Mountain Trail, and Bishop Trail leading south and east, and it braids into two branches about 0.4 miles up (go right on the way up, then take the other branch on the way down later). There is a wide-ranging view from the lookout on the tower (climb with caution).

From the summit, drop 0.1 mile west over ledge outcrops to a junction with the Mount Olga Trail, which forms a 1.5-mile loop down to the campground and back. Go right to follow the north branch 0.7 miles down a west ridge. At the bottom, cross a bridge, climb a short slope to the campground road, and take a left to climb a few hundred feet up through the park to the lower end of the other branch. Take the south branch of the Mount Olga Trail 0.9 miles up the hillside back to the upper junction. Along the way, the trail passes a junction with Shearer Hill Trail on the right and winds through a rocky saddle near the top. From the upper junction, take a right to recross the summit and then return back to the trailhead the way you came.

Optional Extensions   Several trails branch off this loop and head south toward Grant Road and Shearer Hill Road. These include Rim Run, Cross-Mountain Trail, and Bishop Trail to the east and Shearer Hill Trail to the west (the southern part of Shearer Hill Trail is *very* steep). These can be added on as separate out-and-back extensions or combined, with some hilly dirt road miles to connect the southern ends, for a significantly longer loop.

Several miles west, the 2.7-mile-long **Primitive Trail** connects Whites Road near the village of Wilmington with Lake Raponda higher up in the hills. While rough in spots (especially along a somewhat soggy quarter-mile stretch in the middle) and steep for a short stretch near the western end, it is entirely singletrack through scenic forests and generally quite pleasant throughout, though it does not actually go down to the water at the lake. The Primitive Trail is part of the greater Wilmington Trail System, and you can park at either end. Several miles to the east, the **Marlboro Nordic Ski Club**'s network of cross-country ski trails at the campus of the former Marlboro College can be followed in summer. Some are wide and rolling with rough surfaces while others are narrower and more closely resemble regular hiking trails. They can be accessed from a trailhead parking lot on the south side of South Road below the auditorium.

DISTANCE 4 Miles   **TOWN** Wilmington
DIFFICULTY RATING Moderate/Challenging   **TRAIL STYLE** Out-and-Back
TRAIL TYPE Singletrack/Doubletrack   **TOTAL ASCENT** 1,000 Feet

The sharp, 3,425-ft. Haystack Mountain caps the southern end of the prominent north–south trending Deerfield Ridge that looms over the west side of Dover and West Dover. Mount Snow and its ski area are at the northern end. An old road called Deerfield Ridge Trail runs the length of the ridge and may be followed for a longer trek, but at present it is not officially maintained (see the Optional Extension description later in this profile). The Haystack Trail climbs at a mostly steady grade up the south side of Haystack Mountain to the summit. It is infrequently blazed with blue diamond markers. Though it is intermittently rocky and rough, it is fairly easy and straightforward to follow.

DIRECTIONS   From Rte. 9 west of Wilmington, take Haystack Road north for 1.3 miles up the hill. Turn left and go 0.2 miles on Chimney Hill Road. Turn right and go 0.2 miles on Binney Brook Road. Turn left to stay on Binney Brook Road and go 0.2 miles. Turn left again to stay on Binney Brook Road and go 0.4 miles. Turn left to stay on Binney Brook Road one more time and go 0.3 miles. Turn right on Upper Dam Road and go 0.2 miles to the trailhead. Look for the big "HAYSTACK TRAIL" on the sign kiosk as well as a wooden sign on a tree. There is parking for about 10 vehicles along the side of Upper Dam Road. **GPS:** "Mount Haystack, 184 Upper Dam Rd, Wilmington"

TRAIL   From the trailhead, go north up the wide dirt road. The loose rocks slide a bit underfoot here but the footing gets better. Go northwest up and across the slope for 0.5 miles.

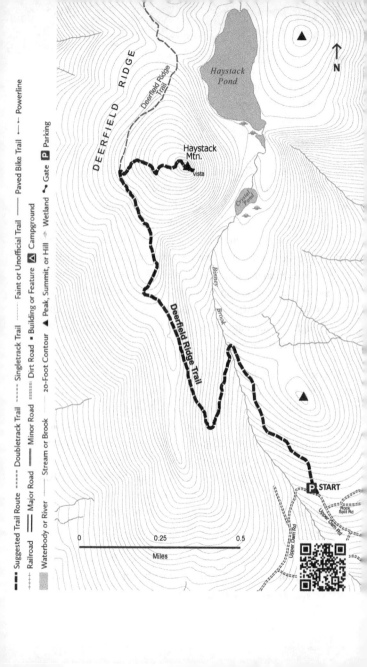

Suggested Trail Route ----- Doubletrack Trail ----- Singletrack Trail .... Faint or Unofficial Trail ---- Paved Bike Trail --- Powerline

++++ Railroad ===== Major Road ======= Minor Road ====== Dirt Road ■ Building or Feature ▲ Campground

Waterbody or River ----- Stream or Brook —— 20-Foot Contour ▲ Peak, Summit, or Hill ✿ Wetland ⌐ Gate P Parking

DEERFIELD RIDGE

Haystack Pond

Deerfield Ridge Trail

Haystack Mtn.
▲ Vista

Crystal Pond

Deerfield Ridge Trail

Binney Brook

N

▲

▲

P START

Rock Split Rd

Upper Dam Rd

Upper Dam Rd

0   0.25   0.5

Miles

At a sign for "Deerfield Ridge Trail No. 306" that says it's 1.4 miles to Haystack Summit, take a left and go southwest across the slope for 0.3 miles on the Haystack Trail, descending slightly to cross a wet area and then rising gently. At a sharp bend to the right, climb northwest at a moderate grade for 0.3 miles. The trail reaches the crest of the mountain's south ridge and levels out slightly for 0.1 mile, then climbs another 0.1 mile to a bend to the right.

Climb at an easy grade for about 0.4 miles. At about 3,100 feet, the trail rises into the dark spruce-fir conifer forest lining the ridgecrest and passes over some exposed bedrock ledges. At a junction, a sign pointing right/east says it's 0.3 miles to the summit. Go right and follow the narrow trail up to the summit of Haystack Mountain where there is a ledge with an east-facing view out over Haystack Pond and beyond. A few hundred feet southeast is another ledge with a slightly less expansive view. To return, head back to the trailhead the way you came up.

Optional Extension From the junction below the summit of Haystack, the Deerfield Ridge Trail leads north along the top of the ridge for about 4 miles to the top of Mount Snow. Overall it's very nice, with fern-lined singletrack leading through a doubletrack-width old road corridor in the woods, but at present there are a few drawbacks: it isn't marked, it's a bit unclear where to go at the northern end, and there are several often-saturated, boggy saddles (though each wet spot has a faint bushwhack path off to the side if you look). There is currently talk of plans to improve this route in the future. *Note that it should not be followed if posted signs say it is closed.*

NEARBY A few miles north, a mix of mountain bike, hiking, and combined hiking/biking trails, amongst the grassy ski trails, lace the eastern slope of **Mount Snow** in West Dover. The **Deerfield Ridge Trail** described above connects Mount Snow to Mount Haystack, though parts are rough, boggy, and remote, and at present the northern end can be hard to find. In the valley below to the east, an unpaved 5-mile portion of the **Valley Trail** leads from just northwest of the Reardon's Crossing pedestrian bridge in the village of Wilmington north to a northern trailhead at Hermitage Club in West Dover, mostly on private or town land. Just north of there, the Valley Trail continues north through nice, recently rehabilitated trail networks east of Handle Road at **Sherwood Forest** and **Crosstown Trails**, where most trails are named after something Robin Hood-ish.

DISTANCE 11 Miles   **TOWN** Stratton
DIFFICULTY RATING Challenging   **TRAIL STYLE** Loop
TRAIL TYPE Singletrack   **TOTAL ASCENT** 2,160 Feet

Towering over the surrounding landscape, 3,918-ft. Stratton Mountain stands as a prominent highlight in the heart of the southern Green Mountains. The suggested route described here combines the Long Trail/Appalachian Trail (LT/AT) and the Stratton Pond Trail for a spectacularly scenic route featuring forested hillsides, a high mountain peak, lovely streams, and pondside views. The route is well marked the whole way and the full loop makes a terrific adventurous trail run option for well-conditioned athletes. Stratton Mountain and Stratton Pond are frequently crowded on weekends in the summer and fall, but are generally more lightly visited during the week. Afterwards, you can cap your workout off with a quick swim in Grout Pond just a few miles to the southeast down a side road, at least during the summer.

DIRECTIONS   From Rte. 100 in West Wardsboro, take Stratton Arlington Road (a.k.a. Kelley Stand Road) west for 8 miles to the Stratton Pond Trail parking area on the right. It is also possible to start this loop from the Stratton Mountain Trailhead about one mile to the east.

GPS: "Stratton Pond Trail Parking, Peru, VT"

TRAIL   The loop starts with a dirt road run from one gravel parking area to another. Follow Stratton Arlington Road about 1 mile due east to the Stratton Mountain Trailhead where the LT/AT crosses. Take a left and follow the white-blazed LT/AT north up into the woods for 1.3 miles, rising at an easy grade up and over a low ridge to a woods road. Cross the road and climb 2.2 miles to the top of Stratton Mountain.

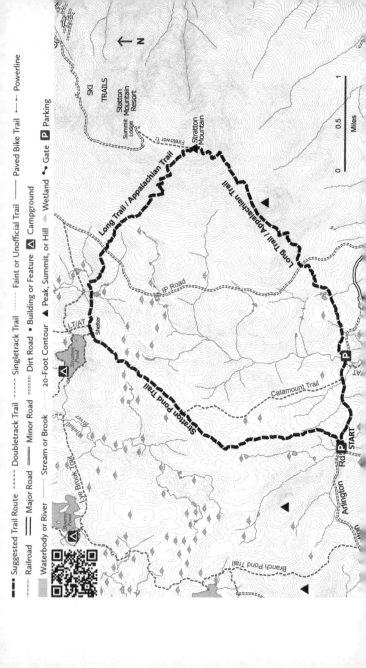

Map Legend

- ▪▪▪ Suggested Trail Route
- ----- Faint or Unofficial Trail
- —— Paved Bike Trail
- ++++ Railroad
- ===== Major Road
- ===== Minor Road
- +--+- Powerline
- ----- Doubletrack Trail
- ----- Singletrack Trail
- ::::::: Dirt Road
- 20-Foot Contour
- ▲ Campground
- ▲ Peak, Summit, or Hill
- ▪ Building or Feature
- Waterbody or River
- —— Stream or Brook
- Wetland
- ⌐ Gate
- P Parking

SKI TRAILS

Stratton Mountain Resort

Summit Mountain Lodge

Firetower Tr.

Stratton Mountain

Long Trail / Appalachian Trail

IP Road

LT/AT

Shelter

Stratton Pond

Stratton Pond Trail

Catamount Trail

Wrinbull's River

Lye Brook Trail

Branch Pond Trail

Arlington Rd

START

P

P

AT

N

0   0.5   1
Miles

The ascent of the mountain is a fun one. There are just enough switchbacks to level the grade to a degree where you can run most of the way, though you'll likely want to hike a few of the steeper bits. For several miles you climb through the forest; it's hardwoods at first, then a mix with conifers, and then finally all spruce-fir conifers near the top.

Stratton Mountain Lookout tower sits in a small clearing at the actual summit; there are magnificent views from up on the fire tower. From the base of the tower, go left at a junction on the LT/AT north.

> *Optional Extension*   You can add a relatively easy extra mile and a
> half to your run with an out-and-back along the Stratton Ridge Trail
> connector path that runs north along the ridge over to the top of
> the chair lift and grassy ski trails at Stratton Mountain Resort. The
> trail dips slightly into a saddle in the middle and crosses a section
> of boardwalks, but for the most part it's quite runnable and fun, and
> the expansive north-facing view is rewarding.

The 1.5-mile descent west from the summit on the LT/AT requires a little bit of trail-running stamina as there are a number of sizable rocks and logs to jump over; it's a good time to work those core muscles. At the base of the mountain, the trail continues west across the rolling landscape for about a mile, crossing several streams and a woods road along the way.

At Stratton Pond you'll need to navigate a small warren of connecting trails and spur paths, including The LT/AT north, Lye Brook Trail, and a shelter spur. Look for the Stratton Pond Trail on the left. You can take time out for a quick swim before lacing back up and heading south for the descent of the Stratton Pond Trail.

The Stratton Pond Trail can be pretty sloppy, with significant muddy patches. But if you hit it on a good day it is easily one of the most fun little stretches of trail running anywhere in New England. For a few miles you roll south along an undulating surface through mixed woods, cross over the Catamount Ski Trail/Winhall Ski Trail about halfway along, and then drop steadily back down to Kelley Stand Road. It's a terrific way to cap off the loop.

> *Alternate Route Options*   For an easy to moderate 7.25-mile run, take the Stratton Pond Trail out and back to the pond. For a more challenging 11.5-mile loop, take Stratton Pond Trail north to the pond, Lye Brook Trail west to Bourne Pond, Branch Pond Trail south past Branch Pond and up to Kelley Stand Road, and Kelley Stand east back down to the trailhead.

NEARBY   About a mile to the south, you can make a fun 2.7-mile run around **Grout Pond** by combining the Pond Loop and Hilltop Trails. The other trails near Grout Pond are managed primarily for winter use and are not generally recommended for running, except for the East Trail/Catamount Trail stretch between the pond and **Somerset Reservoir**. This section of the Catamount Trail to and along the northeastern shore of the reservoir is quite runnable and scenic; however, the Catamount Trail is maintained as a cross-country ski trail, so warm season conditions may vary as you trek further south.

Other good trail runs in the area can be found north and south along the **LT/AT**. A few miles west, the moderately challenging **Branch Pond Trail** makes a 4.7-mile out-and-back run from a small parking area along Kelley Stand Road to a scenic pond. Additionally, several designated hiking trails starting at the **Stratton Mountain Resort** base lodge and Nordic Center climb the peak on ski trails, though they intersect with non-pedestrian trails of the mountain bike park so use caution; bikers have the right of way.

DISTANCE 20 Miles   **TOWN** Jamaica and Londonderry
DIFFICULTY RATING Moderate   **TRAIL STYLE** Out-and-Back
TRAIL TYPE Doubletrack/Singletrack   **TOTAL ASCENT** 1,500 Feet

This section of the West River Trail follows the banks of the West
River between South Londonderry and Jamaica State Park. The trail
is mostly wide and flat, though several miles in the middle follow
narrower, more rugged singletrack up onto the hillside. It passes
through Winhall Brook Campground on a paved road section and
crosses the large Ball Mountain Dam, descending the downstream
side on a set of switchbacks on the side of the dam. The spectacular
scenery includes riverside views, forested streams, and a waterfall.
The route, marked with small purple trail signs along the way, is
described one way following the trail downriver, but there is parking
at both ends and it can be done in either direction (though there is a
fee at Jamaica State Park). There are several side-trail options at Ball
Mountain Dam and the Jamaica State Park end.

DIRECTIONS   From Rte. 100 in South Londonderry, take West River
Street/Town Highway 48 southeast for 0.9 miles. Trailhead parking
is at the end of the dirt road.
GPS: "779 Town Hwy 48 South Londonderry Vermont"

TRAIL   From the end of the dirt road, head southeast on the wide and
flat West River Trail for 0.25 miles. Trace the right side of a wildlife
clearing where there are glimpses of the West River through a thin
woodland strip on the left. At 0.5 miles, cross an open powerline
swath, then continue due south through the woods.
   At 1.8 miles, the trail comes out into the open at Winhall Brook
Campground. Follow the paved campground road/Winhall Station

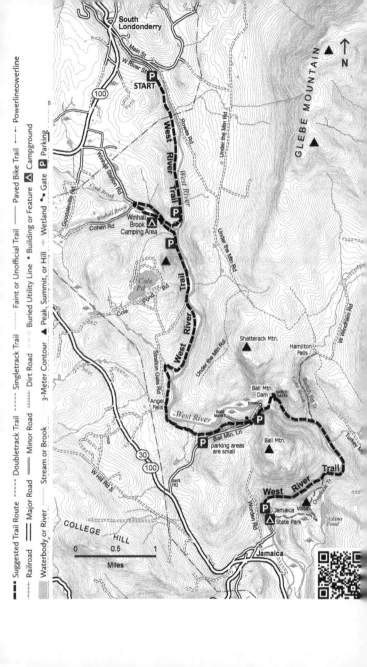

Legend

- ■■■ Suggested Trail Route
- ┼┼┼ Railroad
- ⌁ Waterbody, or River
- ----- Doubletrack Trail
- ═══ Major Road
- ─── Stream or Brook
- ····· Singletrack Trail
- ═══ Minor Road
- ─── Faint or Unofficial Trail
- ▦▦ Dirt Road
- ━━━ Paved Bike Trail
- ···· Buried Utility Line
- ▲ 3-Meter Contour
- ▲ Peak, Summit, or Hill
- ←┼→ Powerline/owerline
- ● Building or Feature
- ▲ Campground
- ⌁ Wetland
- ⌐ Gate
- P Parking

South Londonderry

Main St

W River St

W River St

(100)

START

Roves Rd

West River

West River Trail

Under the Mtn Rd

GLEBE MOUNTAIN

↑ N

Winhall Station Rd

Cook Brook

Goodaleville Rd

Winhall Brook

P

Winhall Brook Camping Area

Cohen Rd

Cole Pd

Pond Rd

Cole

West River Trail

Under the Mtn Rd

Shatterack Mtn.

Hamilton Falls

W Windham Rd

Stratton Gate Rd

Ball Mtn. Dam

switch-backs

tower

Birch Rd Tr

Angel Falls

West River

boat launch

P

Ball Mtn.

Turkey Mtn

P

Ball Mtn. Ln
parking areas
are small

(30)
(100)

W Hill Rd S

park HQ

Warden Rd

Ball Mtn.

West River Trail

Overlook Tr

vista

Adams Pond

P

Jamaica
▲ State Park

COLLEGE HILL

Jamaica

0   0.5   1

Miles

Road southwest and then west for 0.7 miles to a bridge. Turn left and cross the bridge, then immediately take another left and follow the paved road east along the south bank of the brook for 0.7 miles.

Follow the trail back into the woods and go 1.7 miles south along the west bank of the West River. At a marked junction, go right up into the woods at a moderate grade. In 0.2 miles, swing left to cross a bridge, then follow the narrow and more rugged trail south down through the woods and across the slope.

At 5.7 miles from the start, the trail drops down stone steps to cross an unnamed tributary creek in front of Angel Falls, which can be very impressive when water levels in the creek are high. The trail crosses a bridge of laid stones and then climbs the partly open slope on the other side and follows along the wooded hillside above the river. Follow the trail for 1.2 miles as it slowly curves left, well above the river now; it descends to and climbs out of several small tributary stream valleys along this stretch. Bear left at an unmarked junction where an unnamed side trail on the right leads up to Ball Mountain Lane above. In another half mile, stay straight where a brand-new singletrack trail veers up the slope on the right. At a road, bear left on the pavement very briefly and then bear slightly right back onto trail and go a few hundred feet up the hill through the woods to a small parking area along the paved access road just below Ball Mountain Lane.

Bear left at the brown hiker sign and descend 0.25 miles northeast at an easy grade down to the dam. The road turns to dirt at the bottom. Follow the road northeast for 0.2 miles as it climbs diagonally up the west-face side of the dam to the top. Cross over the top and then descend a sharply zig-zagging series of switchbacks known as the Aztec Staircase for 0.2 miles down the east face of the dam. At the bottom, enter the woods and follow the trail 0.15 miles down to the north bank of the river.

Follow the trail above the riverbank for 0.35 miles to a bridge over Cobb Brook. On the other side of the bridge the trail widens to become a dirt road. In 0.15 miles, pass a side trail (Switch Road Trail) leading up to Hamilton Falls on the left. Follow the flat West River Trail for 2 miles as it traces the curves of the river south to Jamaica State Park, passing Overlook Trail on the left and a steep side trail down to a platform above a set of very large boulders called The Dumplings in the river on the right. The trail ends at a playground on the north side of the campground. To return, go back upriver the way you came.

Optional Extension   At the southern end of this route, the blue-blazed Overlook Trail climbs steeply up and over 919-ft. Little Ball Mountain. There is an impressive vista from an open ledge near the top, and the loop adds the variety of significant elevation gain to this suggested route. The southern trailhead in the campground can be somewhat tricky to find (it starts next to the "Hackberry" lean-to shelter), but it's well-signed and the trail is well marked. Doing this loop as a bulb at the south end of the suggested route would add an extra 1.5 miles total.

NEARBY   The entire **West River Trail** between Londonderry and Brattleboro is not contiguous today, but several sections downstream also make excellent running routes. In particular, a flat to very gently sloping, 3.7-mile section between The Marina near the mouth of the West River in Brattleboro and Rice Farm Road in Dummerston features scenic river views and a short (0.2-mile), narrow side branch called Sibosen Trail that ventures out onto a forested floodplain in the **Riverstone Preserve.**

DISTANCE 3.2 Miles   **TOWN** Londonderry

DIFFICULTY RATING Easy/Moderate   **TRAIL STYLE** Loop

TRAIL TYPE Singletrack/Doubletrack   **TOTAL ASCENT** 150 Feet

The blue-blazed Lowell Lake Trail circles a secluded lake and its associated islands and wetlands. The majority is gently rolling singletrack
hiking trail on relatively flat terrain, though some portions follow
dirt roads and wide snowmobile trails. Footing alternates between
good to excellent and somewhat rooty and occasionally muddy. Some
of the highlights include multiple waterside views and picnic sites,
several stands of tall white pine trees, a small boat launch, and a
Revolutionary War–era cemetery. A small portion of the loop southeast
of the lake passes through private property. Lowell Lake State Park is
a very popular destination in the summer. It is a minimally developed
day-use park with limited facilities and parking. The clear and clean
waters make a great way to cool off after a workout on a hot day.

DIRECTIONS   From Londonderry, take Rte. 11 east for 2.9 miles. Turn
left onto Lowell Lake Road and go 0.7 miles north. Turn right on Ice
House Road/Lowell Lake Road (closed in winter) and go 0.2 miles up
to the park. The lot is just past the fee station, above the boat launch.
Parking is tight and there is no alternate parking, so get there early.
GPS: "Lowell Lake State Park, 260 Ice House Road"

TRAIL   From the sign kiosk on the north side of the parking lot, go
north down the wide dirt park road to the boat launch by the lake
where there are great views. Go around a metal gate and follow the
blue-blazed dirt road north for 0.6 miles, passing numerous side
roads down to waterside picnic sites along the way. This portion of
the road passes through the site of a former summer resort camp

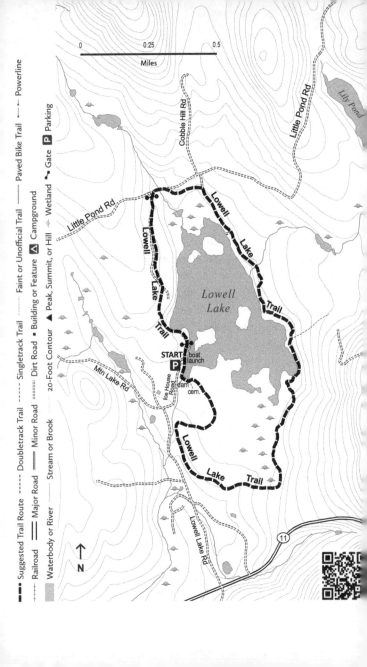

with its old lodge building and various cabins. Bikes are allowed on this portion.

At Little Pond Road, go right and cross a small inlet stream. In about a hundred feet, take a right into the woods on narrow hiking trail; bikes are not allowed beyond this point. In 0.1 mile, take a right on a wide, grassy dirt road. Go south for 0.2 miles to the end of the road.

Go south through the woods along the east side of the lake for 0.4 miles to a short spur path leading west over to a view at the edge of the water. Continue south for 0.2 miles to a junction where an unnamed trail follows blue disc markers up to the left. Bear right and go 0.1 mile down to a view on the southeast side of the lake. Continue south, passing through some boulders and rising slightly up to a ridge. At a trail sign, bear left and climb 0.1 mile south up the pine-covered ridge; this is the steepest part of the loop but it doesn't last long. In about 0.1 mile, bear right on a wider snowmobile corridor and follow it south across the slope for 0.4 miles over several wide bridges and wet areas.

At a "hiking trail" sign, take a right and follow the narrower path west for 0.9 miles as it curves around the south side of the wetland south of the lake. The footing is generally excellent and the grades are easy, and there are numerous small wooden bridges, boardwalks, and gravel cribs over streams and muddy areas along the way.

At the southwest end of the lake, a short side trail leads steeply up to Lowell Lake Cemetery. Take a right to cross the dam, then go right and follow the trail around the western shore past several picnic sites back to the boat launch.

NEARBY A few miles west, the privately owned **Viking Nordic Center** ski area in Londonderry features a network of trails that are excellent for cross-country skiing and snowshoe running.

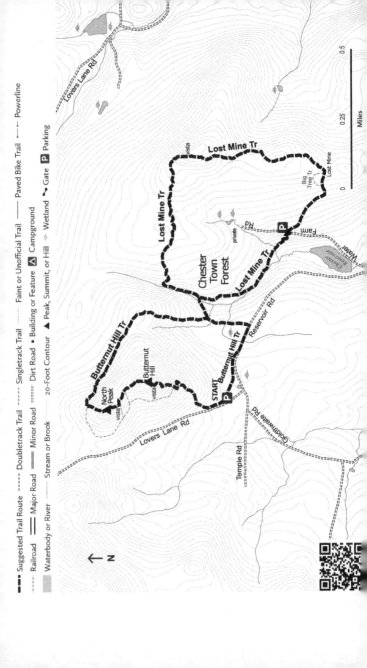

DISTANCE 4.2 Miles   **TOWN** Chester

DIFFICULTY RATING Moderate   **TRAIL STYLE** Figure-8 Loop

TRAIL TYPE Singletrack   **TOTAL ASCENT** 1,020 Feet

This suggested route at Chester Town Forest features a figure-8 of two roughly equal-length, marked trail loops, the Butternut Hill loop and the Lost Mine loop. Each loop is about 2 miles long and the two are linked by a short connector trail in between. The landscape is hilly and rugged, with significant climbs along each loop, and the trail surface is characteristically rocky and rooty with occasional wet spots. There are scenic vistas on each of the two major peaks (Butternut Hill and an unnamed hill to the east), and a number of interesting historic features including an old mine, stone walls, large boulders, a rocky ravine, and several big trees. The forest is primarily northern hardwood with occasional stands of pine and hemlock. There are no facilities at this property and parking space is limited. Dogs are allowed but must be leashed.

DIRECTIONS   From Chester, go 1.8 miles west on Rte. 11. Turn right on Balch Road/Reservoir Road and go 1.6 miles north. Turn right onto Lovers Lane. In 300 feet, the parking area is on the right, next to a green "4900" road marker. Note that there is also another Lovers Lane Road in Chester. A smaller, alternate parking area is available where Lost Mine Trail crosses Water Farm Road.

GPS: "1900 Reservoir Road, Chester" (then go right on Lovers Lane Road)

TRAIL   From the parking area, go north into the woods at a "Chester Town Forest Butternut Hill Trail" sign just past a small wooden bridge. The trail is blazed with white rectangles. The grade is initially gradual as the trail briefly parallels Lovers Lane, but becomes steep and steady as it curves right to climb the south slope of Butternut Hill. At 0.3 miles, just above some switchbacks, pass the first of several faint blue-blazed trails on the left. Stay straight and continue up the hill to a southwest-facing ledge at 0.4 miles where there are two blue chairs and a great view of the surrounding landscape.

Continuing north, cross over the wooded 1,709-ft. summit of the south peak, drop down into a saddle and pass another blue-blazed trail on the left, and climb briefly to a junction with yet another blue-blazed trail on the left where there is a makeshift bench made of branches at a limited vista. Turn right and gently climb to the 1,679-ft. top of the north summit of Butternut Hill at 0.6 miles from the start. Drop down the north side of the hill to a final junction with a blue-blazed trail on the left by a boulder and stone wall.

Optional Extenstion   A rough, lightly maintained blue-blazed trail bypasses both summits of Butternut Hill by traversing the west side of the hill, and there are several short connector trails along the way. This route can be used as a bad-weather route or taken to add extra mileage to the Butternut Hill loop.

Turn sharply right to keep following Butternut Hill loop. After a short, steep descent, traverse southeast along the hillside for 0.4 miles to a ridge. Curve right and descend steadily for 0.3 miles to a junction. Turn left and follow the connector trail 0.1 mile east down the slope and across a low area to a junction.

Take a right and follow the red-blazed Lost Mine Trail counterclockwise, angling diagonally up the hemlock tree-covered slope just below an old woods road. After quickly leveling off below a stony rubble pile, the trail drops for 0.2 miles to a short overlook spur by a stream in a narrow, rocky ravine. Climb diagonally and via switchbacks 0.3 miles east up the slope to Water Farm Road.

Cross the road and continue east up the hill for 0.4 miles to a lower junction with the faint Big Trees trail loop on the left. Stay straight and pass the upper junction in 0.1 mile. The actual old Lost Mine is on the right, with some equipment still visible. Bear left and go 0.5 miles up the south ridge to the high point, crossing a sub summit and saddle along the way. On the north side of the hill is a small vista with a view towards Mount Ascutney, and a stone bench (in memory of Irwin Post). Bear left/west and descend 0.8 miles back down to the start of the Lost Mine Loop; the soft trail surface and gentle downhill grade are especially delightful in this section.

Take a right and follow the Connector Trail back to Butternut Hill Trail. Bear left at the junction and follow the wide, white-blazed trail south across a flat area to Reservoir Road. Take a right and follow the dirt road for 0.1 mile slightly downhill to the west. Veer right off the road onto a grassy snowmobile trail at a green road sign post marked "1464." Follow white blazes gently west up the hill, bearing left at an unsigned junction, to return back to the trailhead.

NEARBY The 1.8-mile **Green Mountain Nature Trail** in Chester makes a lollipop loop up onto a beautiful forested hillside above the high school, with limited views of South Branch Williams River through the trees at the bottom; the trailhead is located near the track.

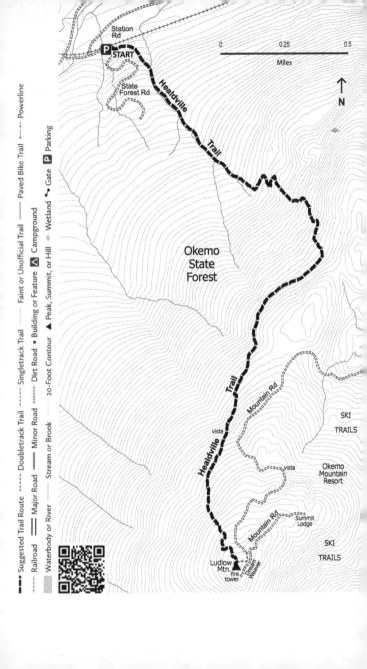

Station Rd

START

State Forest Rd

Healdville Trail

Okemo State Forest

0   0.25   0.5
Miles

N

Mountain Rd

SKI TRAILS

vista

vista

Okemo Mountain Resort

Healdville Trail

Mountain Rd

Summit Lodge

SKI TRAILS

Ludlow Mtn.
fire tower

Dream Weaver

Suggested Trail Route ···· Doubletrack Trail ----- Singletrack Trail ----- Faint or Unofficial Trail ——— Paved Bike Trail ——— Powerline
+++++ Railroad ——— Major Road ≡≡≡≡ Minor Road ∷∷∷∷ Dirt Road ■ Building or Feature ▲ Campground
——— Waterbody or River ——— Stream or Brook ——— 20-Foot Contour ▲ Peak, Summit, or Hill ⬩ Wetland ⟍ Gate 🅿 Parking

DISTANCE 6 Miles **TOWN** Ludlow

DIFFICULTY RATING Moderate/Challenging **TRAIL STYLE** Out-and-Back

TRAIL TYPE Singletrack **TOTAL ASCENT** 1,890 Feet

Located entirely within Okemo State Forest, the 3-mile-long Healdville Trail climbs to the wooded summit of 3,320-ft. Ludlow Mountain. The trail, built in the early 1990s by the Vermont Youth Conservation Corps (VYCC), is marked with rectangular blue blazes and is easy to follow. In the first mile, it criss-crosses the Catamount Trail (a cross-country ski route marked with blue arrow signs) several times and makes a sustained, moderately steep ascent. The second mile rises at a gentler grade and features several nice switchbacks and cross-slope traverses. The third mile is somewhat steeper again and passes several vistas. There are excellent views from a fire tower at the summit. On the descent, all three miles are one hundred percent runnable and extremely enjoyable.

DIRECTIONS From Ludlow, take Rte. 103 north for 4.5 miles. Turn left on Station Road and go 0.7 miles southwest. Just after crossing the railroad tracks, turn left on State Forest Road and go about a few hundred feet east to the Healdville Trail parking lot, which holds about ten vehicles.

GPS: "Healdville Trail Mount Holly" (then go east a few hundred feet to parking)

TRAIL From the map kiosk at the trailhead, pass between two boulders and take the wide Healdville Trail east across the hillside above the railroad tracks. In about 0.2 miles, after crossing several streams on wooden bridges, the trail swings right and begins a sustained, 0.7-mile climb straight up the slope at a moderate grade to the left of a brook. The trail is somewhat rocky in places here, and it also crosses the Catamount Trail at several junctions; make sure to stay on Healdville Trail.

At a curve to the left, the trail climbs a series of switchbacks at a slightly gentler grade for 0.6 miles through a cove of semi-rich hardwood forest on the northwest side of the mountain. After bearing right at the top of one final switchback, the trail angles south across a plateau on the slope for 0.5 miles, crossing a few seepy spots on rocks along the way.

At the 2-mile mark, the trail begins climbing the slope at a steady, moderate grade. Then at about 2.5 miles, after passing a small clearing with an excellent west-facing vista, it steepens even more and ascends a series of switchbacks for 0.3 miles to a set of mossy, fern-covered rock ledges. It then climbs another 0.1 mile to an old stone chimney (the remains of a former ranger cabin) in a flat spot and a junction just beyond. The Healdville Trail technically ends here. The trail to the left leads down to the top of the Okemo Mountain ski area and access road.

Take a right and climb 0.1 mile on the Okemo Summit Trail to the fire tower. You can climb to the top where there is a 360-degree view of the surrounding south-central Vermont landscape. To return to the trailhead, go back down to the Healdville Trail the way you came up.

Optional Extension   It's possible to take a combination of trail and dirt road from the top of the mountain over to the Okemo Mountain Resort's Summit Lodge, which is open seasonally for hot chocolate and other treats. From the junction just below the fire tower (where a sign says "Mt Road Parking Lot 0.3"), follow the Okemo Summit Trail northeast 0.1 mile down to Mountain Road. Take a right on the wide Mountain Road and then immediately bear left at a junction where the Dream Weaver ski trail leads right and then pass by some buildings. Go 0.3 miles northeast on Mountain Road, which gently descends 0.3 miles to the lodge, staying left where several ski trails drop down to the right. Total round-trip distance for this extension is about 0.8 miles.

NEARBY A few miles east, a mile-long trail explores three primary sets of cascades at **Buttermilk Falls** in Ludlow; multiple swimming holes here makes a great place to cool off after a run on a hot day. Just south of Buttermilk Falls, two new trails leave from Okemo Mountain Resort's Jackson Gore Inn; the 0.5-mile **Jackson Gore Falls Trail** and the 1.2-mile **Sawmill Loop**. Both of these short trails are of moderate to challenging difficulty. Several miles to the northeast, the **Echo Lake Vista Trail** makes a moderately difficult, 1.1-mile lollipop loop to a vista on the lower slopes of Blueberry Hill above Camp Plymouth State Park.

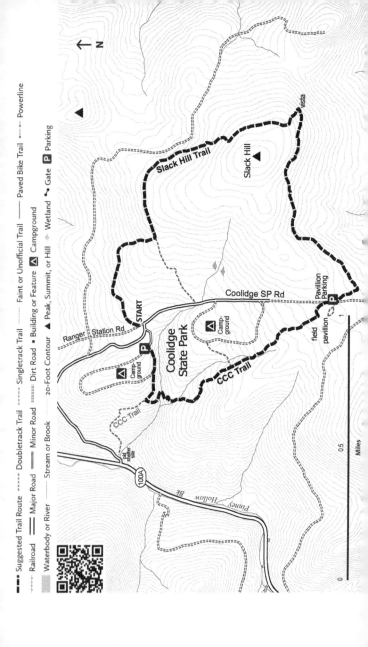

← N

Suggested Trail Route ----- Doubletrack Trail ····· Singletrack Trail ------ Faint or Unofficial Trail —— Paved Bike Trail —•— Powerline
+++ Railroad —— Major Road ≡≡≡ Minor Road ∷∷∷ Dirt Road • Building or Feature ▲ Campground
—— Waterbody or River —— Stream or Brook — 20-Foot Contour ▲ Peak, Summit, or Hill ❀ Wetland ❧ Gate 🅟 Parking

Slack Hill Trail

Slack Hill ▲

vista

▲

Ranger Station Rd

START

🅟

Coolidge SP Rd

Coolidge State Park

▲ Camp-ground

Pavillion Parking

🅟

field
pavillion

CCC Trail

▲ Camp-ground

CCC Trail

pic shelter site

100A

Putney Hollow Bk

Miles
0   0.5   1

DISTANCE 4 Miles   **TOWN** Plymouth
DIFFICULTY RATING Moderate   **TRAIL STYLE** Loop
TRAIL TYPE Singletrack   **TOTAL ASCENT** 760 Feet

While not one of the highest or most prominent peaks in its immediate vicinity, 2,174-ft. Slack Hill nevertheless is one of the highest
points in Coolidge State Park (a subunit of the larger Coolidge State
Forest). The relatively high-elevation park features many developed yet
rustic amenities and facilities that make it a favorite for campers and
day-use visitors alike. The suggested route described here combines
the park's two most popular hiking trails, Slack Hill Trail and CCC
Trail, into a moderately difficult but generally quite easy to follow
loop around the park that includes deep woods, scenic vistas, and a
steep stream valley. The entire loop is marked with blue blazes and
there are signs at all junctions. Recent tree harvests to prevent the
spread of invasive insects have thinned the woods considerably in
many areas here, ash trees in particular, but the trail corridors have
been well maintained. A fee is charged to enter and use the park
during the operating season, and the road into the park is closed in
winter, but the loop can also be accessed from a small parking area
at the bottom of the hill.

DIRECTIONS   From Woodstock, go 8 miles west on Rte. 4. Turn left
on Rte. 100A and go 3.7 miles. Turn left on Ranger Station Road and
go 0.7 miles up the hill on the park road. At the ranger station, turn
right and go 200 feet on Coolidge State Park Road. Hiker parking is
along the edge of the road along the field. Ranger Station Road is
closed in winter.
GPS: "855 Coolidge State Park Road"

TRAIL   From the Slack Hill Trail sign next to the park office, go east up the hill at an easy grade into a recently harvested woodland of mixed hardwood trees. After a brief descent at 0.2 miles, climb at a moderate then slightly steeper grade to a junction at 0.5 miles. The connector trail to the right drops steadily for 0.3 miles down to the park road above the office.

Turn left/west and follow the trail 0.4 miles as it traces a level southward curve to the right across the slope. Then climb at a moderate grade for 0.5 miles, cross over the east side of the hill, and drop briefly down to a vista clearing on the southeast side of the hill at 1.5 miles from the start where there is a log bench with a view of Mount Ascutney on the far horizon.

Go west from the vista, following the rolling trail across the slope for 0.5 miles before descending steadily for 0.3 miles. Curve to the right and climb 0.1 mile (see figure 7) to an upper trailhead and day-use parking area along Coolidge State Park Road. Cross the road to the other side where an accessible gravel trail leads over to the Bradley Hill picnic pavilion at the top of an open field.

To the right, look for the CCC Trail sign about 100 feet north down the road. Take the CCC Trail 0.1 mile through the woods to the open field, then bear right to follow the mowed path along the upper edge of the field downhill for 0.2 miles. Follow the trail into the woods and downhill at a moderate grade for about 0.3 miles to a junction where a side trail leads right over to a tenting area. Continue straight on the trail down the hill for 0.4 miles or so. Curve sharply right at the top of a bluff and drop steeply down into a ravine.

Cross the small brook at the bottom of the gorge, then climb steadily for 0.2 miles up the hemlock-covered slope on the other side. At a junction where the CCC Trail continues downhill to the left, go right and follow the spur trail up to the lean-to campground loop road. Go right on the road back to the trailhead.

Optional Extension or Approach   The lower end of the CCC Trail begins at a trailhead next to an old picnic shelter site right at the base of the paved park road near Rte. 100A. This can be used as an alternate approach if the park road is closed, or for a slightly longer and more difficult lollipop version of the loop. It is a steep half-mile climb mostly along an old fire road to the junction with the spur trail leading up to the lean-to campground road.

NEARBY   The **Shrewsbury Peak** site is located several miles to the northwest (see next site).

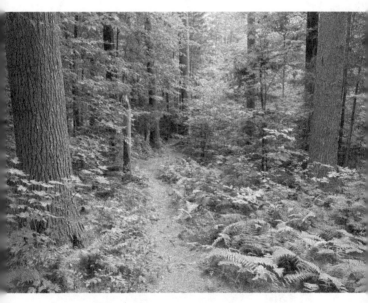

FIGURE 7. Slack Hill Trail in Coolidge State Park in Plymouth.

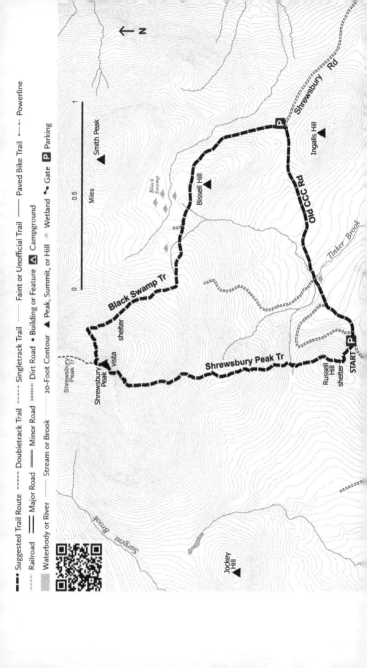

Suggested Trail Route ···· Doubletrack Trail ----- Singletrack Trail ······ Faint or Unofficial Trail —— Paved Bike Trail +-+ Powerline

++++ Railroad ═══ Major Road ══════ Minor Road ══════ Dirt Road ▪ Building or Feature ▲ Campground

▒ Waterbody or River —— Stream or Brook ──── 20-Foot Contour ▲ Peak, Summit, or Hill ❀ Wetland ◟ Gate ☐ Parking

← N

Smith Peak ▲

Black Swamp

Bissell Hill ▲

Ingalls Hill ▲

Shrewsbury Rd

Old CCC Rd

Tinker Brook

Black Swamp Tr

shelter

Shrewsbury Peak Tr

Shrewsbury Peak
vista

shelter

Russell Hill
shelter

START ☐

Shrewsbury Peak Tr

Sargent Brook

Jockey Hill ▲

Miles

0   0.5   1

DISTANCE 3.7 Miles   **TOWN** Shrewsbury

DIFFICULTY RATING Moderate/Challenging   **TRAIL STYLE** Loop

TRAIL TYPE Singletrack   **TOTAL ASCENT** 1,590 Feet

Shrewsbury Peak is a relatively high (3,381 feet) mountain capping the south end of the Coolidge Range ridge, which includes Mendon, Little Killington, Killington, and Pico peaks further north. This route makes a loop by linking the Shrewsbury Peak Trail, Black Swamp Trail, and Old CCC Road. On the ascent, the grade alternates back-and-forth between steep and moderate, with occasional flats and even a short downhill now and then. But mostly it's moderately steep. The descent is gentler, and includes several long, smooth stretches and a section along a dirt road.

DIRECTIONS   From Rte. 4 between Woodstock and Killington, go 3.2 miles south on Rte. 100. Turn right/west on Shrewsbury/Old CCC Road (dirt) and go up and over a ridge for 3.2 miles to the parking area on the right. This road is closed in winter.
GPS: "Shrewsbury Peak Trailhead Old CCC Road"

TRAIL   From a sign kiosk at the edge of the Russell Hill parking lot, the blue-blazed trail enters a stand of cedar trees and rises a few hundred feet up the hill to the remains of some Civilian Conservation Corps-era construction, including a stone pavilion chimney and a wishing well. From the well, climb steeply north for 0.1 mile to a lean-to shelter. Pass the shelter at 0.2 miles, cross over the broad, wooded crest of 2,530-ft. Russell Hill (consider this the low front-range precursor to Shrewsbury Peak), then drop down the north side of the hill to a junction with the Catamount Trail along a woods road at 0.4 miles.

Drop steeply into a dark, narrow, rocky gully at 0.5 miles, then climb out the other side just as steeply. At 0.7 miles cross over a grassy woods road. At 0.8 miles, the trail levels out slightly, bears left, and continues gradually climbing diagonally up the side of the slope through northern hardwood forest until it comes out into a glade-like area at 1.3 miles, which it then pushes up into. Not long after that, the trail abruptly rises out of the hardwoods entirely and enters a zone of dense spruce and fir trees with occasional white birch. Rain or shine, the deep-green mossy understory here seems to glow.

Entering the Shrewsbury Peak Natural Area, climb very steeply north up through the conifer forest to the ridge just south of the top. Continue northeast at a slightly easier grade, past a small rocky outcrop with a limited view to the south, to the summit at 1.7 miles where there is a small outcrop with extensive views to the south and east.

From the summit, descend north a few hundred feet to a faint spur path leading northwest to a limited vista. After that, drop briefly down to a trail junction in a mossy col and take a right.

Follow the blue-blazed Black Swamp Trail down to the east at a comparatively easy grade. In 0.3 miles, pass the Shrewsbury Peak Shelter lean-to on the right. From the shelter, gradually descend southeast along the grade of an old woods road for 0.9 miles to a clearing. Black Swamp, an important bear-feeding area in spring, lies in a basin to the left.

Go straight across the clearing, climb briefly at a gentle grade along the north side of Bissell Hill, then follow the wide, grassy Black Swamp Road for 0.6 miles as it descends through hardwood forests to a gate just before a parking area along Old CCC Road. To complete the loop, go right on Old CCC Road and follow it 1.3 miles west back to the Russell Hill parking area, dropping downhill for about a mile and then climbing slightly at the end.

Optional Extensions   From the junction just north of the Shrewsbury Peak summit, the Black Swamp Trail continues north for 1.9 miles across the ridge to a junction with the Long Trail/Appalachian Trail (LT/AT) just below the top of Little Killington Peak. Nearly the entire length is through boreal spruce-fir forest except for a short dip down into a mountain pass. From there you can take the LT/AT two more miles north to Cooper Lodge and Killington Peak. The final few tenths of a mile on the spur trail to the summit are very steep. Total round-trip extra distance to the top of Killington is just under 8 miles.

NEARBY A few miles to the west, the **LT/AT** leads about 5 miles northeast from a trailhead along the Cold River up to Killington Peak. Though parking is challenging and the route is long, this is one of the easiest ways to climb Killington. The **Bucklin Trail** that climbs about 4 miles up from Brewers Corner to the west is also nice, and shorter, but it is steeper and it tends to be more crowded.

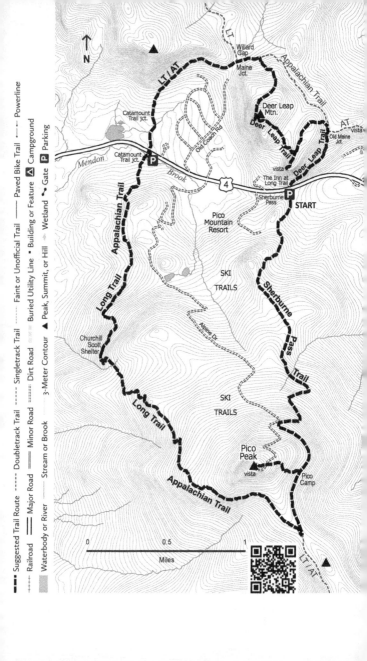

N

LT

Willard Gap

Maine Jct.

LT / AT

Appalachian Trail

Deer Leap Mtn.

Deer Leap Trail

AT

vista

Old Maine Jct.

Catamount Trail Jct.

Old Coach Rd

Deer Leap Trail

Catamount Trail Jct.

P

vista

Mendon

Brook

The Inn at Long Trail

4

Sherburne Pass

P

START

Appalachian Trail

Pico Mountain Resort

Long Trail

SKI TRAILS

Sherburne Pass Trail

Alpine Dr.

Churchill Scott Shelter

SKI TRAILS

Long Trail

Pico Peak

vista

Pico Camp

Appalachian Trail

LT / AT

- ▪ Suggested Trail Route
- ┊ ┊ ┊
- ┼┼┼ Railroad
- ═══ Major Road
- ——— Waterbody or River
- ╌╌╌ Doubletrack Trail
- ╌╌╌ Singletrack Trail
- ══ Minor Road
- ═══ Stream or Brook
- ········ Faint or Unofficial Trail
- ╌╌╌ Dirt Road
- ━━━ Powerline
- ▪ ▪ ▪ ▪ Buried Utility Line
- ▲ Peak, Summit, or Hill
- • Building or Feature
- ✦ Wetland
- ▲ Campground
- ╲ Gate
- P Parking
- vista

0   0.5   1
Miles

DISTANCE 10 Miles   **TOWN** Killington and Mendon

DIFFICULTY RATING Challenging   **TRAIL STYLE** Loop

TRAIL TYPE Singletrack   **TOTAL ASCENT** 3,035 Feet

The Pico Loop is a classic Vermont trail run. Incorporating a relatively new section of the Long Trail/Appalachian Trail (LT/AT) and the old route on what is now the Sherburne Pass Trail as well as a northern excursion to Deer Leap Mountain, it features a wealth of amazing scenery, rich green forest, challenging terrain, and gorgeous trails. It can be started from either of two trailheads along Rte. 4 and is fun in both directions. The summit of Pico Peak is reached by a steep but worthwhile side-trail excursion along the main loop.

DIRECTIONS   From Rte. 7 in Rutland, take Rte. 4 east for 9 miles to the top of Sherburne Pass. From Rte. I-89 near White River Junction, take Rte. 4 west for 31 miles to Sherburne Pass. The parking lot is on the south side of the road across from Inn at Long Trail (a great place for trail adventurers to stay or eat at). An alternate parking area is located at the LT/AT crossing about half a mile west down the hill on the south side of Rte. 4.

GPS: "Sherburne Pass"

TRAIL   From the trailhead kiosk on the south/upper side of the parking lot, head south into the woods on the blue-blazed Sherburne Pass Trail along the grade of an old road. At 0.1 mile, bear right at a fork with a hiker's register. Climb steadily for 0.4 miles. About half a mile into the ascent, portions of the trail more or less parallel the deeply eroded trench of the former, older route.

At about 0.5 miles, you can see light from the westernmost of the Pico ski trails through the trees to the right. Before reaching them, though, the trail swings slightly left at a level bench and continues to climb through the woods just to the west. After a mostly level stretch with smooth footing, the trail begins to climb at a relatively gentle grade via a series of long switchbacks through mixed hardwood conifer forest, with the occasional large old birch. There are the usual rocks and roots.

At 1.9 miles, the trail reaches an open ski trail, swings left and climbs it briefly, then reenters the woods on the left. After the ski trail the footing gets significantly more rugged with a lot of slippery rocks and roots. It's more level, though, and even occasionally descends slightly as the trail traverses its way around the eastern side of Pico Peak through distinctly boreal forest. The roots are gnarly here, the rocks a bit mossier, and everything somewhat slippery, but it's altogether gorgeous. At 2.3 miles you arrive at Pico Camp Shelter.

From the shelter, the blue-blazed Pico Link trail climbs, quite steeply at times, for 0.4 miles to the top, crossing an open ski area access road with great views of Killington on the way. After climbing steeply through increasingly stunted trees, it crosses another dirt road then finally comes out at and follows an open ski trail to the top. Follow it to the top of the chairlift, then look for the blue blazes signifying the little path around the back of the operator hut. The actual top of the mountain is marked by a small, grassy pile of stones amongst the windswept conifer trees. Descend Pico Link back to the shelter.

Go south across the slope for 0.25 miles, cross a wide dirt road (Killington-Pico Connector), then go another 0.25 miles to a junction with the Long Trail/Appalachian Trail (LT/AT).

Optional Extension From this junction, follow the LT/AT south as it rolls along the ridge past Rams Head Mountain and Snowdon Peak and up to the summit of 4,242-ft. Killington Peak, the second highest mountain in Vermont. This section of trail is remarkably beautiful as it passes through dark, mossy spruce-fir forest, and the footing is excellent most of the way. The grade is generally gentle to moderate, but the final climb to the exposed top of the mountain is extremely steep and not particularly runnable.

Turn right and follow the LT/AT northwest across the slope for 0.4 miles back towards Pico. Swing left and descend steadily for 1.3 miles to a junction with a spur leading left to Churchill Scott Shelter, passing back into northern hardwood forest along the way. Bear right and continue descending north at a gentle grade with occasional short climbs for 1.7 miles down to a junction with the Catamount Trail.

Go right and cross a bridge over Mendon Brook, then reach a junction amongst roadside shrubs where a short spur leads right/east over to a parking area. Go left and carefully cross busy Rte. 4, then head back into the woods at a trail sign on the north side of the road.

After crossing a wet area on bog bridges and then crossing a stream, pass a junction where the Catamount Trail leads left/west at 0.2 miles from the road, and climb northeast through open woodland for 0.5 miles at a steady, moderate grade. When the trail levels off, go 0.25 miles east across the slope to Maine Junction (formerly Willard Gap). At this important point, the Long Trail leads left to go north while the Appalachian Trail continues straight ahead (and a path on the right is marked with a "this is not a trail" sign). Go straight and follow the AT 0.1 mile east up to a junction.

Alternate Route If you don't want to climb up and over Deer Leap Mountain, continue straight. The next quarter to half-mile stretch of the LT/AT is quite runnable and scenic, and you can still make an out-and-back trip to the view at Deer Leap Rock from the next junction.

Turn right and take the Deer Leap Trail steeply for 0.5 miles up the north side of Deer Leap Mountain. After cresting a ridge and leveling off, pass just west of the 2,782-ft. wooded summit and then drop steeply down ledges for 0.3 miles to a saddle. Climb steeply up the other side and scramble up a rocky ledge to a junction. Take a right and go 0.1 mile through conifer forest south down to 2,526-ft. Deer Leap Rock where there is a spectacular view to the south from a prominent rock outcrop.

Climb back up to the junction, then take a right to follow the blue-blazed Deer Leap Trail northeast for 0.3 miles northeast across and down the mountain to a junction. Turn right and follow the AT 0.1 mile south to another junction (formerly the original Maine Junction). The AT leads left/east down to Gifford Woods State Park from here. Bear right and follow Deer Leap Trail steeply down the slope to the south to a trailhead next to Inn at Long Trail at the top of Sherburne Pass. Carefully re-cross Rte. 4 back to the start.

NEARBY Just to the south, **Killington Peak** can also be reached by a 7.2-mile round-trip ascent of the heavily used Bucklin Trail from Wheelerville Road in Mendon.

DISTANCE 4.5 Miles   **TOWN** Mendon and Chittenden
DIFFICULTY RATING Moderate   **TRAIL STYLE** Out-and-Back
TRAIL TYPE Singletrack   **TOTAL ASCENT** 1,500 Feet

Blue Ridge Mountain caps a prominent rise along the western escarpment of the Green Mountains south of Chittenden Reservoir and north
of Rte. 4. Though the mountain features several wooded, trailless
peaks further north, the blue-blazed Canty Trail provides access to
the mountain's high point at its 3,248-ft. southernmost peak. This
route consists of a fairly straightforward out-and-back trip, with
short side-trail spurs to a pretty waterfall and scenic vista ledge. It
starts out fairly level and easy, but the grade and terrain get gradually
steeper and rougher the further upslope you go.

DIRECTIONS   From Rte. 7 in Rutland, take Rte. 4 east for 6 miles.
Bear left onto Old Turnpike Road and go 1 mile northeast. There is
limited parking for several vehicles in a gravel pull-off on the left
side of the road.

GPS: "Blue Ridge Mountain Trailhead"

TRAIL   From the "Canty Trail" sign at the trailhead, follow the trail
west into the woods. After descending to a small brook, the trail
gently undulates up and down through the woods, bypassing a few
wet areas and crossing several small streams along the way. At 0.7
miles, cross a more sizable stream on cobbles; this may be tricky in
the spring or after heavy rains.

Climb the stone steps up the bank on the other side of the stream,
then veer right onto a wider section at a signpost with blue arrows
(the old route goes left). Follow the trail north across a level area.
Soon after, the grade steepens and the footing becomes more rugged

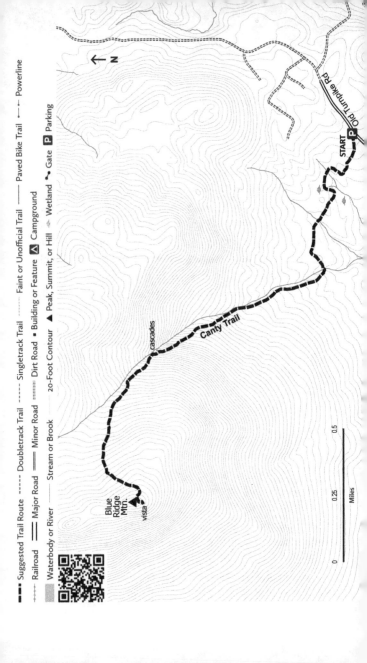

Legend:

- ■■■ Suggested Trail Route
- ----- Doubletrack Trail
- ----- Singletrack Trail
- ········· Faint or Unofficial Trail
- —— Paved Bike Trail
- ┼┼┼┼ Railroad
- ══ Major Road
- ═══ Minor Road
- ┈┈┈ Dirt Road
- ┈┈┈ 20-Foot Contour
- •┈• Powerline
- —— Waterbody or River
- —— Stream or Brook
- • Building or Feature
- ▲ Campground
- ▲ Peak, Summit, or Hill
- ⇔ Wetland
- ⚲ Gate
- **P** Parking

N →

START

Old Turnpike Rd

P

Canty Trail

cascades

Blue Ridge Mtn.

vista

0   0.25   0.5

Miles

as you ascend along the west side of Sawyer Brook. Climb steadily northwest through northern hardwoods for just over half a mile.

At 1.5 miles, go right at a very short spur trail leading down to a set of cascades. Back on the main trail, continue climbing up past the upper cascades, then veer slightly left away from the brook. The grade lessens some as you enter mossy conifer forest near the summit.

At 2.2 miles, go right at a junction and continue following the blue-blazed trail to the top where there is a limited view to the east from a small rock outcrop. Back down at the junction, follow the spur path 0.1 mile west down to a more expansive vista at a ledge with a view southwest over Rutland to the Taconic Range beyond. To return, retrace your route back to the trailhead.

NEARBY A few miles north, a combination of rough trails and woods roads rings **Chittenden Reservoir** for an 8.5-mile loop (water access not allowed), and the **Long Trail** traverses the high ridge east of the lake. About 8 miles south, the 3.3-mile **Bald Mountain Trail** lollipop loop summits 2,074-ft. Bald Mountain (not bald) at Aitken State Forest in Mendon; this moderate route features several nice views but is somewhat poorly marked.

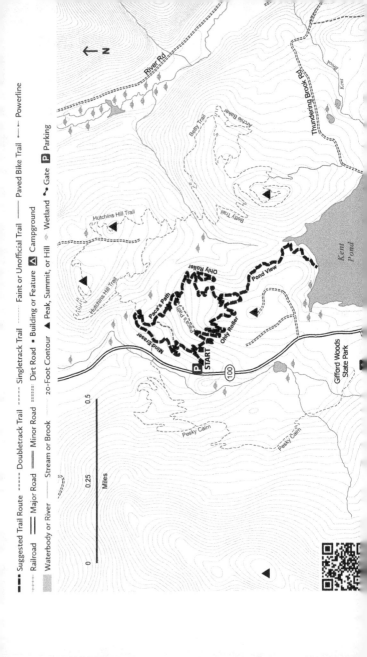

← N

━━ Suggested Trail Route ‑‑‑‑‑ Doubletrack Trail ‑‑‑‑‑ Faint or Unofficial Trail ━━━ Paved Bike Trail ‑+‑ Powerline
++++ Railroad ━━ Major Road ═════ Minor Road ░░░░ Dirt Road • Building or Feature ▲ Campground
━━ Waterbody or River ━━━ Stream or Brook ─── 20-Foot Contour ▲ Peak, Summit, or Hill ⟡ Wetland ⟍ Gate 🅿 Parking

River Rd

Kent Brook

Thundering Brook Rd

Archie Baker

Betty Trail

Betty Trail

Hutchins Hill Trail

Hutchins Hill Trail

Only Roller

Paca's Path

Paca's Path

Mind Eraser

START

🅿

Only Roller

Pond View

Kent Pond

100

Gifford Woods State Park

Pesky Calm

Pesky Calm

0   0.25   0.5

Miles

DISTANCE 2.6 Miles   **TOWN** Killington

DIFFICULTY RATING Moderate   **TRAIL STYLE** Lollipop Loop

TRAIL TYPE Singletrack   **TOTAL ASCENT** 260 Feet

Sherburne Trails hosts a network of well-built marked loop trails that were designed for mountain biking but are open to multiple non-motorized uses. A relatively new trail system, it has quickly become a popular spot for hikers and dog walkers as well as bikers; please respect all other users. The trails feature sharp, banked turns and occasional technical rock challenges, but they are easy to follow and the footing is excellent throughout. The suggested loop here simply follows the main loop through the part on Forest Service land, but there are also two other similarly fun, but slightly more challenging loops over and around hills on private land to the north and east; please obey any posted signs if you connect to either of them. Dogs are allowed but must be leashed.

DIRECTIONS   From the junction with Rte. 4, take Rte. 100 north for 1.3 miles to the Green Mountain National Forest Sherburne Trails Trailhead parking lot on the right.

GPS: "Sherburne Trails"

TRAIL   From the map kiosk above the parking lot at the trailhead, go east up the entrance trail into the woods. Climb at a gentle grade up a set of switchbacks to a fork at jct. 1. Bear right onto Paca's Path and climb gently up more switchbacks for 0.3 miles to jct. 5.

Leaving Paca's Path, take a right onto Ohly Roller and go 0.4 miles up more switchbacks to the top of the hill. Weave around several boulders and exposed bedrock ledges and then drop slightly down to jct. 6.

Optional Extension   Take a right and follow Pond View trail gently down the south side of the hill for 0.5 miles to the north edge of Kent Pond. Total round-trip distance is 1 mile.

From jct. 6, follow Ohly Roller for 0.7 miles as it winds north down the hillside via a long sequence of banked curves and switchbacks to jct. 4. Take a right onto Paca's Path and continue down the north side of the hill for 0.3 miles to jct. 3. Take a right on Mind Eraser and descend another 0.1 mile to an unmarked junction where an unsigned trail (Sherburne Connector) leads right.

Optional Extension   Take a right and follow Sherburne Connector (signed on the other side) across a boardwalk bridge over a low area and then 0.2 miles up to a junction marking the start of Hutching Hill loop trail. Take a right. The Hutching Hill trail immediately splits into easier and harder branches; go right for the easier one (the harder one is intended for experienced bikers). Follow this trail 0.5 miles east along and then down the slope to a junction with a trail leading right to yet another trail loop system. Go left and follow Hutching Hill trail for 1.4 miles, climbing up and over the hill several times on swoopy switchbacks, back to the start of the loop. Then take the Sherburne Connector back. Total round-trip distance is about 2.4 miles.

From the unmarked junction on Mind Eraser, go southeast along the base of the hill for 0.2 miles to another unmarked junction where a trail leads right/west over to cross Rte. 100 to link up with Pesky Cairn Trail and Gifford Woods State Park to the south. Bear left and follow Mind Eraser around the slope and up to jct. 2. Take a right and follow Mind Eraser south for 0.1 mile back to jct. 1, then drop down the entrance trail to the parking area.

NEARBY   A few miles south, the 1.5-mile Kent Brook Trail/Gifford Woods Loop encircles the campground at **Gifford Woods State Park**

in Killington. This site can be linked to directly from Sherburne Trails by carefully crossing Rte. 100 and following Pesky Cairn Trail about 2 miles south. The new Sherburner Trail is particularly excellent for running here; it is a unidirectional 3-mile loop on the west side of Pesky Cairn. The **Appalachian Trail (AT)** also passes through the park after descending from Deer Leap Mountain and before making its way around the south shore of Kent Pond (a rare flat section) towards **Thundering Brook Falls** in Killington (where there is a section of wheelchair-accessible boardwalk). East of Killington, the AT begins a long section of climbing to and passing through remote woods on the way east towards Woodstock and beyond.

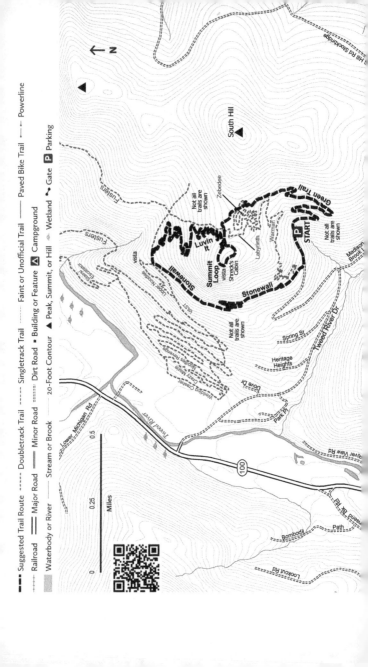

DISTANCE 3.3 Miles   **TOWN** Pittsfield and Stockbridge
DIFFICULTY RATING Moderate/Challenging   **TRAIL STYLE** Loop
TRAIL TYPE Singletrack   **TOTAL ASCENT** 420 Feet

Green Mountain Trails hosts a 25-mile network of extremely well built and maintained trails that are open to mountain biking, running, hiking, and snowshoeing. The trail system covers the northwest slope of 2,074-ft. South Hill, and there are a wide variety of surface types, difficulty levels, and distances. One flowy descent from the summit is over six miles long from start to finish. Several highly technical trails are left unmapped on purpose. This suggested loop, a short one to keep it relatively simple, incorporates a sampling of some of the best routes for running but represents just a fraction of the possibilities at the site. It is possible to enter the network from below at Amee Farm barn (look for trail signs and a map kiosk), but the bridge over the Tweed River is currently out so it requires a stream crossing. Note that trails may be closed during unusually wet conditions or large events. Several grueling competitions take place here every year, in both summer and winter, including ultramarathons, trail races, snowshoe races, and adventure races, and the empowering and inspiring spirit of digging deep to rise to the challenge is strong.

DIRECTIONS   From Rte. 4 in Killington, take Rte. 100 north for 7.1 miles. Turn right on Town Highway 32/Tweed River Drive and go 1 mile east up the hill to a junction with Madison Brook Lane. Take a hard left to stay on Tweed River Drive and go 0.35 miles to a sharp turn. Take a right to stay on Tweed River Drive and go 0.35 miles up a rougher section of road to the parking area; it can be helpful to have a high-clearance vehicle for the final 0.35 miles.

TRAIL   From the trailhead at the top of Tweed River Drive, take the wide trail up the grassy hillside above a stone cabin (called Fiona's) to a sign marking the start of Green Trail. Staying straight where a trail called Yonder leads right, follow the green-blazed (and occasionally green arrowed and yellow-diamond markered) Green Trail up the hillside via a series of long, gentle switchbacks for 0.7 miles. There are several marked and unmarked junctions along the way.

At a junction where a sign points left to Warman and Labyrinth trails and another sign points straight ahead to Shrek's Cabin, stay straight on Green Trail. Go 0.2 miles north, climbing a few more switchbacks, to a confusing set of junctions. Stay right at a first junction where Zebedee trail leads left, then immediately cross two intersections with a lobe of Zebedee, pass a junction with Over Yonder on the right, and finally bear right at a junction with the other end of Zebedee. Just stay on Green Trail at all of the junctions. Continue following Green Trail for another 0.1 mile to its upper end at an intersection where Fusters leads right and Labyrinth leads left.

> *Optional Extension*   The aforementioned Zebedee trail winds crazily around, down, and back up a small section of the upper hillside for nearly a mile, ending very close to where it begins. The switchback turns are legion, and it's easy to feel turned around, but the bottom line is that this trail is very fun to run.

Go straight for 0.1 mile to a junction. Go straight to follow Summit Loop up and around to the left for 0.15 miles to an open meadow, passing the upper ends of the Stone Steps hiking trail and Devil's Throat (a downhill-only bike trail) on the right. A stone hut called Shrek's Cabin sits in the clearing, where there are excellent westward views of the mountains on the other side of the valley. Beyond the cabin, drop 0.1 mile down Summit Loop to a junction, passing a side trail called Roland's Run on the right along the way.

At the intersection, bear left for a few feet and then turn right on the (occasionally) white-blazed Luvin' It trail (marked as "Lubbin' Eet" on one sign) and descend via dozens of tight switchbacks for about 1.1 miles to an intersection. Along the way you'll pass and/or cross numerous other trails, including Bubba and connector links over to Fusters just to the right and Devil's Throat just to the left. At the intersection, a short trek to the right on Stonewall leads to a scenic vista called Pittsfield Overlook.

Take a left and follow the purple-blazed Stonewall trail at a nearly level grade south across the steeply sloped hillside for 0.8 miles. About two thirds of the way along, a short way past a solitary trio of narrow switchbacks up a steep pitch, Stonewall crosses over a very impressive section of the Stone Steps hiking trail, which at this spot seems to consist entirely of large, hand-placed stone steps. From the intersection with the lower end of Warman trail, drop down the southward extension of Stonewall a few hundred feet out to Tweed River Road, then take a left and climb the road back up to the parking area.

Optional Extensions Numerous other trails are great for trail running here, including Upper Noodles, Noodles Revenge, Rabbit Hole, Fusters, and Stairs/Escalator, among others. The Stone Steps hiking trail also makes a highly taxing hill workout.

NEARBY A few miles west across the Tweed River and up Michigan Road along the West Branch of Tweed Brook, a network of double-track paths, woods roads, and snowmobile corridors leads up onto **Bloodroot Mountain** and **Thousand Acre Hill** and intersect with the **Long Trail** above Chittenden Reservoir. A few miles north, the **Contest Trail** in Pittsfield makes a 6.7-mile lollipop loop on old woods roads and features amazing views from Mayo Meadow; it starts from a trailhead on Old Liberty Road.

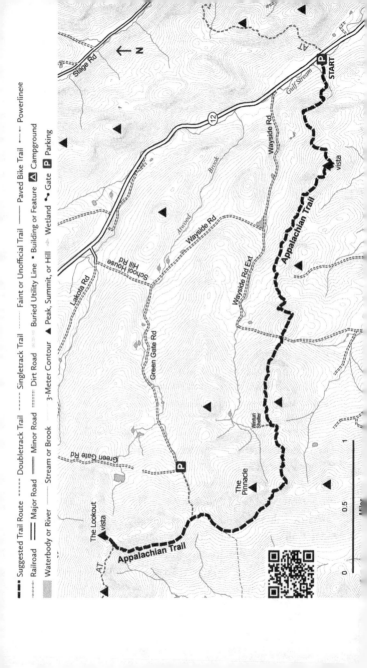

Suggested Trail Route ···· Doubletrack Trail ----- Singletrack Trail ···· Faint or Unofficial Trail —— Paved Bike Trail ⊢—⊣ Powerline
++++ Railroad —— Major Road —— Minor Road ===== Dirt Road ----- Buried Utility Line • Building or Feature ▲ Campground
▬ Waterbody or River —— Stream or Brook —— 3-Meter Contour ▲ Peak, Summit, or Hill ⌐⌐ Gate ↰ Wetland 🅿 Parking

N

Stage Rd

Gulf Stream

START 🅿

Wayside Rd

Appalachian Trail

vista

12

Atwood Brook

Wayside Rd

School House Hill Rd

Lakota Rd

Green Gate Rd

Wayside Rd Ext

Appalachian Trail

Winturi Shelter

Green Gate Rd

🅿

The Lookout
vista

AT

The Pinnacle

0   0.5   1
Miles

DISTANCE 11.4 Miles   **TOWN** Woodstock
DIFFICULTY RATING Moderate   **TRAIL STYLE** Out-and-Back
TRAIL TYPE Singletrack   **TOTAL ASCENT** 2,830 Feet

On its long way north to Mount Katahdin in Maine, the Appalachian Trail (AT) abruptly diverges from the path of the Long Trail in Vermont at Deer Leap Mountain and forges eastward on a 43-mile trek across the middle of the state to the Connecticut River and New Hampshire. Despite leaving the Green Mountains behind, the elevation profile is anything but level as the trail crosses several sizable hills and ridges, and dips down into multiple river valleys along the way, sometimes quite steeply. This out-and-back section features significant elevation gain but it is spread out over a lengthy distance, and a few sections near the upper end are actually close to level. It climbs from hill to hill along a ridge and tops out at a pair of low mountains. The footing is generally excellent, though of course there are the usual occasional rocky and rooty patches throughout. Highlights include a view from The Lookout, pleasant stretches of trail through classic northern hardwood forest, and narrow ribbons of trail through scenic hillside meadows.

DIRECTIONS   From Exit 1 off of I-89, go 10 miles west on Rte. 4 to Woodstock. Turn right on Rte. 12 and go north for 2.8 miles. Turn left into a short gravel drive (may be rough). The small trailhead parking lot is just below the level of the road.
GPS: "AT Trailhead Woodstock Vermont"

TRAIL   From the trailhead, cross Gulf Stream on a sturdy wooden bridge, pass through a gate designed to keep livestock in, and go west up the hillside on the white-blazed AT. The trail crosses in and out of fields as it climbs, sometimes alongside grazing cows. At one point it crosses over an electric fence; be particularly mindful here. After ascending through an open meadow at 0.3 miles (see figure 8), the trail swings right and climbs steeply north up a wooded ridge alongside a narrow ravine to the top of an unnamed hill at 0.5 miles.

Drop down the north side of the hill, then bear west and rise steadily for 0.6 miles to a clearing at the top of the next hill. There is a view of Mount Ascutney here. Reenter the woods, descend slightly, then climb 0.2 miles to the top of another partly bald hill. From here, continue west for 1.3 miles through hardwood forest, dropping slightly then gradually rising to the top of another hill. Then descend 0.1 mile to a saddle and cross over Wayside Road Extension (essentially just a woods road here).

Climb at a moderate grade for 0.3 miles, then traverse the north side of the ridge for 0.4 miles to a junction with a spur trail leading right down to Winnturi Shelter. Bear left and climb for 0.6 miles at increasingly steeper but never "steep" grades to the top of a small conifer-covered knoll called Sawyer's Hill. Cross over the peak and drop 0.1 mile down to a saddle, then bear left beneath the ledges of The Pinnacle and descend 0.2 miles. Here, begin a 0.7-mile, nearly level traverse of the west slope of the mountain, eventually along the grade of an old road, to a junction (rising slightly just before the end).

At a junction where a blue-blazed side trail drops down an old road to the right (Lookout Farm Road), bear left on the AT. Go 0.6 miles northwest through birch glades and hardwoods along the west side of the ridge, rising and falling a few times and passing a spring along the way. Then start a steep, 0.2-mile climb to a junction.

Go right and follow the spur trail for 0.1 mile up to Luce's Lookout, a private cabin near the 2,435-ft. top of a small spruce-capped peak called The Lookout. There's a view from ledges in front of the cabin, but the unique highlight here is the widow's walk. A very steep wooden ladder on the outside of the building climbs to a small platform on the roof where the view is even better. Needless to say, use extreme caution when using both the ladder and the platform.

Return to the trailhead the way you came, or descend the Lookout

Trail to Green Gate Road and make your way back down via several miles of mostly dirt roads (Green Gate, Wayside, and Rte. 12).

NEARBY On the other side of Rte. 12 at this trailhead, it's a 1.6-mile climb, quite steep at first, on the **Appalachian Trail** (AT) up to 1,522-ft. **Dana Hill** where there is an open sloping meadow with great views just before the summit. To the east, the AT generally stays at lower elevations, topping out on a shoulder of 1,962-ft. **Thistle Hill** in Pomfret, though there are still a number of steep climbs and descents into and out of valleys, and finding parking can be a surprising challenge along some of the road crossings. The sections around **Cloudland Road** and **Joe Ranger Road** are especially nice for trail running, particularly the short parts that pass through scenic open meadows and fields on idyllic-looking hillsides. About ten miles north, there is a small network of pedestrian-only loop trails at **Amity Pond Natural Area State Park** in northern Pomfret.

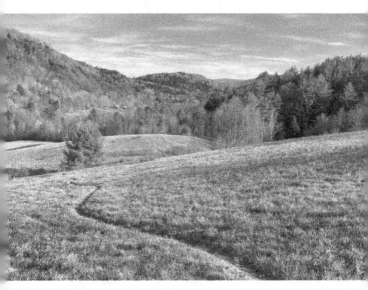

FIGURE 8. The Appalachian Trail near Woodstock.

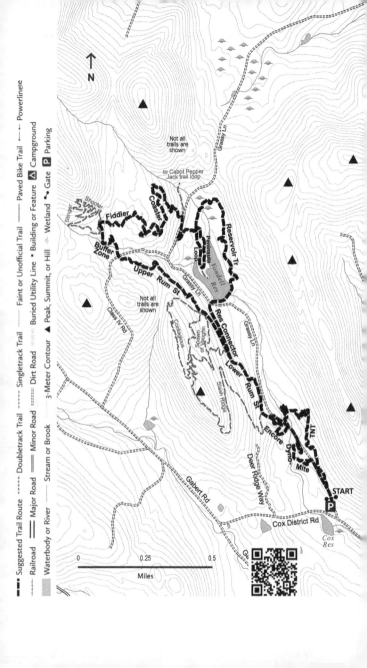

Legend:

- Suggested Trail Route
- Railroad
- Waterbody or River
- Doubletrack Trail
- Minor Road
- Stream or Brook
- Singletrack Trail
- Dirt Road
- 3-Meter Contour
- Faint or Unofficial Trail
- Buried Utility Line
- ▲ Peak, Summit, or Hill
- Paved Bike Trail
- Building or Feature
- Gate
- Powerline
- ▲ Campground
- Wetland
- 🅿 Parking

↑ N

Not all trails are shown

to Cabot Pepper Jack trail loop

Shooter

Fiddler

Coaster

Reservoir Trl

Peninsula Loop

Wendell Res

Buffer Zone

Upper Rum St

Grassy Ln

Class IV Rd

Not all trails are shown

Res Connector

Contagious

Spasm

Slash Ridge

Grassy Ln

Lower Rum St

Encore

Dyno

Mite

TNT

Deer Ridge Way

Gabert Rd

START

🅿

Cox District Rd

Cox Res

0   0.25   0.5

Miles

DISTANCE 5.5 Miles   **TOWN** Woodstock

DIFFICULTY RATING Moderate   **TRAIL STYLE** Figure-8 Loop

TRAIL TYPE Singletrack   **TOTAL ASCENT** 570 Feet

Woodstock's Aqueduct Trails is a relatively new web of interwoven multi-use paths around Vondell Reservoir up in the hills west of town. While the trails are not blazed, they are easy to follow, with generally excellent footing throughout, and all intersections are well-marked with wooden posts. There are many wooden bridges and boardwalks that cross over wet areas and sensitive habitats. As with all multi-use trail systems, please be respectful of other users and kindly offer people the right-of-way when you encounter them or they come up behind you. There are no summit vistas or ledges, but the reservoir itself is scenic, the forests are pleasant, and the trails pass through several open fields. The land is owned by the Woodstock Aqueduct Company and the terrific trails are maintained by the Woodstock Area Mountain Bike Association.

DIRECTIONS   From Exit 1 off of I-89, go 10 miles west on Rte. 4 to Woodstock. Then take Rte. 4 west for 2 miles. Turn right on Cox District Road and go 0.8 miles. Turn right on Grassy Lane. The parking lot is 230 feet ahead on the left.

GPS: "Woodstock Aqueduct Company Trails, 23111 Cox District Road"

TRAIL   From the trailhead, go north up the wide dirt road known as Grassy Lane. In 0.1 mile, at the crest of the rise, bear right at a junction onto TNT trail and follow it for 0.7 miles as it gently winds up, around, and down the hillside. Just before rejoining Grassy Lane, it crosses a wooden bridge and rises slightly. Take a right and go 0.1 mile northwest on Grassy Lane to a field.

Bear left into the field and look for the start of Lower Rum Street trail at the far end. Bear right onto that trail and follow it 0.3 miles gently uphill to a junction. Bear right onto Reservoir Connector and follow it 0.2 miles north across a level area to an intersection.

Cross over Grassy Lane and take Reservoir trail 0.1 mile east across the grassy berm at the south end of Vondell Reservoir. Enter the woods on the far side and follow Reservoir trail for 0.6 miles. It undulates along the west slope of a ridge and then curves left through a forested cove north of the reservoir, eventually heading south.

At a fork, stay straight then immediately bear left at another fork to follow the Peninsula trail loop counterclockwise around a wooded peninsula at the north end of the pond. Back at the two forks, go straight and then immediately bear right back onto Reservoir trail and go 0.1 mile to a junction just below Grassy Lane.

Take a right onto Coaster and head north, crossing over Grassy Lane soon after. Follow Coaster up the hill, passing a junction with a trail leading over to the new Cabot Loop on the right, and follow it for 0.8 miles up and around the hillside to a grassy landing at the upper end of a logging road. Coaster is slightly steeper and more challenging than the other trails so far. Bear left on the grassy road and immediately bear right back into the woods to take Fiddler 0.1 mile west to an intersection with Buffer Zone and Shooter trails.

Take a left and follow Buffer Zone downhill for 0.2 miles to a Class IV road. Cross the road and follow Upper Rum Street 0.2 miles downhill. Cross over Spawn Connector and follow Middle Rum Street across the slope for 0.2 miles to an intersection. Take a right and follow Lower Spawn of Vaughn for 0.4 miles up, across, and down the hill to a junction with Lower Rum Street (you can also just continue on Middle Rum for another 0.2 easy miles instead of swooping around on Lower Spawn). From here, return back to the trailhead the way you came in but also tacking on a few extra swoopy bits with the short Encore (0.2 miles) and Dyn-o-mite (0.3 miles) handles on the right/west side of Grassy Lane near the end.

Optional Extensions   Several more challenging trail loops can be taken north and west of the reservoir. These include the highly technical Stinger/Shooter combo mentioned above as well as Contagious and Slash Ridge up above Rum Run. There is also a brand-new loop trail north of Coaster called Cabot Pepper Jack.

NEARBY The western trailhead for **Marsh-Billings-Rockefeller National Historical Park** is located only a few miles east along Prosper Road. From there you can make an easy 2.5-mile loop up to **The Pogue** on Prosper Trail and North Ridge Loop, or make a moderately difficult 1.5-mile round-trip climb up **West Ridge Trail** to the top of the unnamed hill west of the pond. You can also link to the network of multi-use trails of Vermont Land Trust's **King Farm** from here via Maple Trail or White Pine Trail.

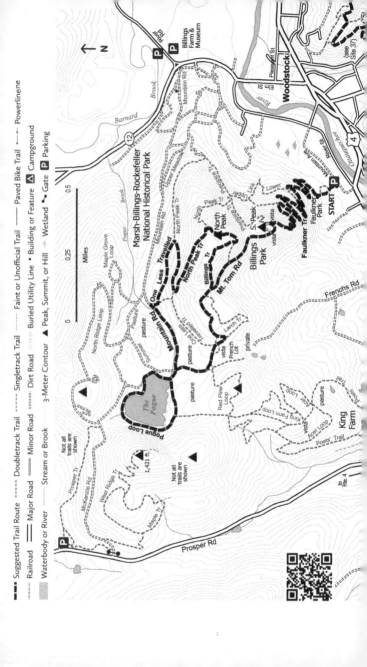

Legend

- ▪▪▪ Suggested Trail Route
- +++ Railroad
- ═══ Major Road
- ===== Minor Road
- ----- Doubletrack Trail
- ----- Singletrack Trail
- ═══ Dirt Road
- ⌇⌇⌇⌇ Buried Utility Line
- ── Stream or Brook
- ----- Faint or Unofficial Trail
- ─── Paved Bike Trail
- ▲ Peak, Summit, or Hill
- ── 3-Meter Contour
- ─── Powerline
- ▲ Building or Feature
- ⌇ Wetland
- ↘ Gate
- △ Campground
- P Parking

N ↑

Marsh-Billings-Rockefeller National Historical Park

Billings Farm & Museum

Woodstock

The Pogue

Pogue Loop

1,421 ft.

Not all trails are shown

Not all trails are shown

King Farm

Prosper Rd

to Rte. 4

Mountain Rd

One Less Traveller

North Peak Tr

Billings Tr

Mt. Tom Rd

Billings Park

Faulkner Park

Faulkner Trail

START

North Peak

S. Peak

vista

vista

vista

vista

Frenchs Rd

private

French Lot

Larch Tr

Red Pine Loop

Acer Loop

King Farm Loop

Poets' Loop

Poets' Trail

Prosper Tr

McKenzie Rd

West Ridge Tr

Maple Tr

North Ridge Loop

Maple Grove Loop

Upper Meadow

Mountain Rd

North Peak Tr

pasture

pasture

pasture

pasture

pasture

Barnard Brook

Pogue Brook

River St

Elm St

Mountain Ave

Ottauquechee River

12

4

Miles

0   0.25   0.5

DISTANCE 6.5 Miles   **TOWN** Woodstock

DIFFICULTY RATING Moderate   **TRAIL STYLE** Lollipop Loop

TRAIL TYPE Singletrack   **TOTAL ASCENT** 800 Feet

This spectacular site combines trails on properties owned and managed by the National Park Service and the Town of Woodstock. Vermont's only national park, the Marsh-Billings-Rockefeller National Historical Park, was created in 1992 when the former owners bequeathed it to the federal government. The Pogue, a small man-made pond ringed by hills up in the center of the park, is a clear highlight and focal point of any trip to the park. Trails of all kinds crisscross the entire property, and posted poetry excerpts by Robert Frost can be found scattered throughout the park. Note that the trails are groomed for cross-country skiing in winter and are closed to other uses (besides snowshoeing in designated areas). Dogs are welcome but must be leashed (leashes are even provided at one trailhead). Bordering the historical park to the south are two smaller ones, Billings Park and Faulkner Park. The north peak of Mount Tom and the wild Precipice Trail are two notable features of Billings Park, which is owned by the Town of Woodstock, and the Faulkner Trail to the views on the south peak of Mount Tom is a clear highlight of Faulkner Park, managed by Faulkner Trust. The excellent trail networks of all three parks blend more or less seamlessly on the ground, as do the trails at Vermont Land Trust's King Farm to the southwest.

DIRECTIONS   From Exit 1 off of I-89, go 10 miles west on Rte. 4 to Woodstock. Turn right on Mountain Avenue, cross the Ottauquechee River through a one-lane covered bridge, and go 0.2 miles to Faulkner Park on the right where there is roadside parking.

GPS: "Faulkner Park Woodstock"

From Woodstock, go north on Rte. 12 for 0.4 miles, then bear right onto Old River Road and then take an immediate left into the overflow parking lot for the park at 65 Old River Road across the street from the main parking area; from there, paved pedestrian connector pathways link to a trailhead by the carriage barn. From there it is 1.6 miles up wide carriage trails to The Pogue.

TRAIL At the Faulkner Park field, look for the map sign kiosk at the end of the paved path. Go into the woods on the stone-lined, crushed gravel pathway that is the start of the Faulkner Trail. Follow the many long switchbacks of the extremely well-maintained Faulkner Trail at a gentle grade for 1.5 miles to a junction just below the 1,250-ft. summit of the south peak of Mount Tom. Please do not take any of the erosion-enhancing switchback cutoffs (why would any runner *want* to?). On the way up, you'll pass multiple junctions with link trails on the right and pass numerous boulders, rock ledges, benches, and stone bridges, steps, and embankments. The trail is always well-marked and easy to follow. Near the top, the grade increases and it gets rockier, and there is even a steel cable railing to assist you up an almost technical scramble on a ledge section with a steep drop-off to the right.

At the top there is a lookout view south out over the village and the Ottauquechee Valley. Go left a few hundred feet on the wide Mount Tom Road to an expansive west-facing vista towards the Green Mountains. Follow the road 0.9 miles northwest to a junction with Mountain Road just below The Pogue. It first descends to a narrow col between the south and north peaks, then curves left and passes junctions and intersections with many trails on both the left and right. The final stretch descends along the east side of an open hillside field.

Turn left and take Mountain Road 0.1 mile up to The Pogue. From a junction, take the mostly flat 0.85-mile Pogue Lakeside Trail loop around the pond (see figure 9). Whichever direction you choose, the scenery is undeniably spectacular.

Descend east on Mountain Road carriage path for 0.25 miles

through the upper part of a narrow stream valley. Take a sharp right and climb steeply up the slightly narrower One Less Travelled Trail. The next few junctions are somewhat tricky. Turn left at an unmarked junction with an old trail just up from Mountain Road. Go 0.3 miles east across the slope. Take a right and go west across the slope on a 0.1-mile section where One Less Travelled Trail and North Peak Trail share the same route. Then turn left and follow North Peak Trail up and east across the slope for 0.3 miles to a junction.

Take a right and follow Billings Trail 0.1 mile up towards and just east of the 1,359-ft. summit of Mount Tom's North Peak. Billings Trail then meanders 0.3 miles around the south side of the summit, passing a shortcut down to the left and eventually descending west to a junction with Mount Tom Road. Take a right and return back

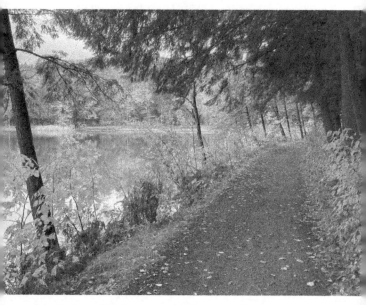

FIGURE 9. Trail around The Pogue at Marsh-Billings-Rockefeller National Historical Park.

down the mountain via the Faulkner Trail, taking special care on the ledgy part at the top.

> *Optional Extensions*   The trails of these parks and conserved proper-
> ties range from wide, flat carriage trails to steep, rugged hiking trails
> with iron safety rails. Any of them are fun for trail running, though
> it's probably best to carefully walk some parts of the Precipice Trail.
> Notable other trails to explore include North Ridge Loop, West
> Ridge Trail, King Farm Loop, Red Pine Loop, the Larch Trail, and
> Upper and Lower Link trails.

NEARBY   Across town to the southeast, **Mount Peg** features a small but scenic network of pedestrian-only trails to a 1,090-ft. peak with terrific views above an open hillside meadow, as well as a much larger system of adjacent mountain bike, snowshoe, and cross-country ski trails on private land just to the south.

DISTANCE 2 Miles **TOWN** Woodstock

DIFFICULTY RATING Moderate **TRAIL STYLE** Loop

TRAIL TYPE Singletrack **TOTAL ASCENT** 300 Feet

A large and complicated trail network covers much of the north–south ridge that rises prominently above the southeast side of Woodstock. While the true high points (Mount Charlie, Baylies Hill, and Garvin Hill) lie further south, the north end of the ridge is capped by the 1,090-ft. sub-summit of Mount Peg where there is a terrific vista at an open hillside meadow. The town manages Mount Peg Park on the lower northwest side of the mountain, while the rest of the ridge is owned and managed by the Woodstock Inn and other private landowners. The popular trails within the public park are pedestrian-only but the remainder are multi-use, primarily for mountain biking, and snowshoe and cross-country ski activities in the winter. Passes must be purchased to use the private trails. Most of the trails are well graded and well maintained, and generally feature excellent footing. This short route is great if you only have limited time or just want a quick workout with a great view, and it is a good choice for beginner trail runners looking to gain some experience with climbing and descending.

DIRECTIONS From Exit 1 off of I-89, go 10 miles west on Rte. 4 to Woodstock. Turn left on High Street and go 0.2 miles south. Turn left on Golf Avenue and go 0.1 mile southeast. There is a small parking on the left at the base of Billing Place (essentially a driveway). If this lot is full, there is also public parking available nearby in town. **GPS:** "Billings Place Woodstock" or "Billings Park and Trails"

TRAIL From the parking lot, go a hundred feet up Billing Place to the trailhead map kiosk. Start out on the Mount Peg Summit Trail.

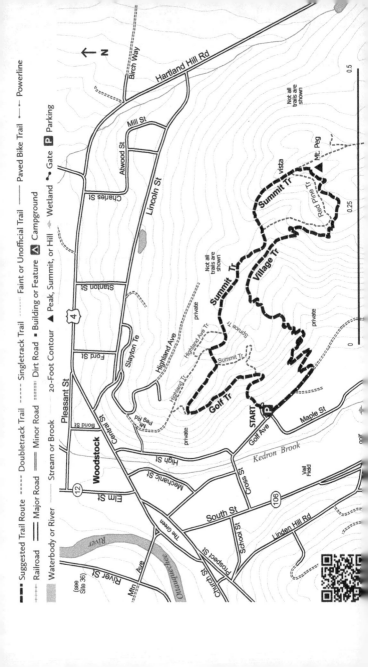

In 0.1 mile, go left at a junction and follow Golf Trail diagonally northwest up the side of the ridge at a gentle grade for 0.2 miles. Passing a junction on the left, the trail curves sharply right and continues another 0.2 miles up to an upper junction with Summit Trail. Turn left and go steeply for a few hundred feet up to a junction with a bench. Turn right and follow Summit Trail east along the ridge for about 0.2 miles. Pass a junction with Spruce Trail on the right and continue east for 0.2 miles to an intersection. Cross over Lincoln Street Link and emerge out into an open field. Pass a junction with the lower end of Red Pine Trail and follow Summit Trail the rest of the way to the top of Mount Peg, rising through an open field as you climb. There are benches and a picnic table at the top.

From the vista, look for the three-forked intersection of trails heading south. Take the middle one, Village Trail. Follow Village Trail as it swoops back and forth many times for 1 mile down the west side of the hill to Golf Avenue. This well-constructed new trail is wide, flowy, and very fun to run down. Be particularly mindful of and friendly to other trail users here; Village Trail was built as a mountain bike route to and from the village and is well used both up and down. To return to the parking lot, turn right and go 0.1 mile northwest on Golf Avenue.

Optional Extensions   There are several other short trails in the Mount Peg Park network that can be combined to add extra mileage, including Spruce Trail, Summit Trail, Highland Avenue Trail, Red Pine Trail, and several links.

NEARBY   About 8 miles east on Rte. 4, there are several short (and very popular) hiking trails in and around the impressive Quechee Gorge at **Quechee State Park** in Hartford.

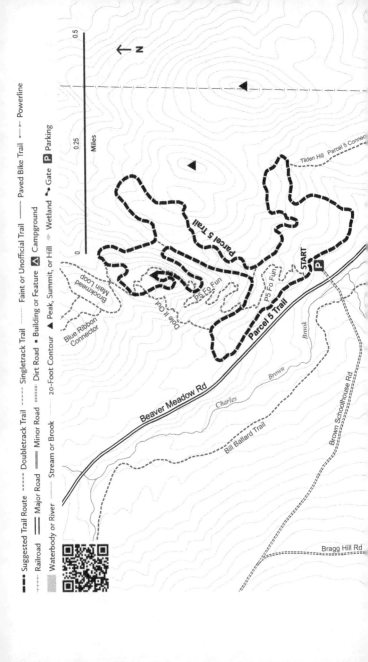

DISTANCE 3.2 Miles   **TOWN** Norwich

DIFFICULTY RATING Moderate   **TRAIL STYLE** Loop

TRAIL TYPE Doubletrack/Singletrack   **TOTAL ASCENT** 680 Feet

Parcel 5 is the name of this site as well as the name of the wide, carriage-trail-like loop that winds around it. Footing and trail markings are excellent the entire way, though some parts are steep enough to bump the difficulty rating up to moderate. Along the way there are several short connectors to shorten or add on extra loops. Weaving across and alongside the main Parcel 5 trail in the western part of the site are a couple of more challenging singletrack mountain-bike trail options called P5 Fo Fun and Dole It Out. In addition to the signage, maps are posted at many of the major intersections.

DIRECTIONS   From I-89 at White River Junction, take I-91 north for 4.6 miles to Exit 13. Take Rte. 5 north through Norwich for 0.7 miles. Turn left on Beaver Meadow Road and go 2.4 miles northwest. Look for a small "Parcel 5" sign on the right. The spacious parking area is up a short gravel driveway on the right.

GPS: "Parcel 5 Norwich"

TRAIL   The Parcel 5 Trail is intended to be followed one way. From the trailhead, go left through a small grassy area above the parking lot and enter the woods to the north. After passing the lower end of the narrow P5 Fo Fun, the trail rolls up and down along the hillside for a while and then curves right and passes the lower end of Dole It Out at 0.5 miles. In 0.1 mile, P5 Fo Fun crosses this route at an intersection. In another 0.1 mile there's a junction where a short interior connector path leads right.

Bear left and begin climbing up the hill at a steady grade. In 0.2 miles, pass another link on the right and curve sharply left up a steep curve. Re-cross P5 Fo Fun in 0.2 miles and then climb another 0.25 miles up to the top of this hill. Drop slightly and cross an intersection with Dole It Out, then reach a fork where a wide path leads downhill to a small field from which a spur trail leads north into Brookmead Conservation Area.

Go right at the fork, pass an easy-to-miss singletrack spur on the left leading to Brookmead, and follow Parcel 5 Trail for 1.9 miles down and around the hillside back to the trailhead, passing several interior connector trail links on the right and crossing intersections with a few steep old roads that weave through near the bottom. The overall trend is downhill in this latter half, though there are also a few relatively short uphill climbs.

Optional Extensions The Brookmead Conservation Area trail system abuts Parcel 5 just to the north; there are 4.2 miles of blue-blazed trail options there overall. Across Beaver Meadow Road and a bridge over Charles Brown Brook just to the southwest of Parcel 5, the Bill Ballard Trail (named for a former biology professor at Dartmouth College) crosses Brown Schoolhouse Road and provides many miles of very nice, moderately challenging terrain. Highlights to the north along Upper Ballard include a section through a ravine called "Grand Canyon" and the 0.4-mile Converse Loop. A challenging 6–7-mile loop, fun in either direction, can be created by combining Parcel 5, Brookmead, Blue Ribbon Connector, and Bill Ballard Trail. A challenging extension of that loop could tack on the 8.4-mile round-trip trek up to the top of Gile Mountain on the Blue Ribbon Trail.

NEARBY Norwich has a remarkable network of often interconnected trails all over town. Directly connected to Parcel 5 are the **Bill Ballard Trail** (partitioned into Upper Ballard and Lower Ballard) and the **Converse Loop**, the **Blue Ribbon Trail** (which links to Gile Mountain), and **Brookmead Conservation Area**.

A few miles north, the very popular Gile Mountain Trail leads 0.7 miles to a fire tower at the summit of 1,854-ft. **Gile Mountain**. A 1.1-mile bike trail crosses back and forth over the main hiking trail, providing a longer and gentler way of ascending or descending. Both trails are impressively well constructed and easy to follow. The parking lot fills up fast on weekends and during leaf season. One town north, there's a nice network of multi-use trails at **Thetford Hill State Park**.

About two miles south, on the other side of a ridge above Beaver Meadow Road, **Cossingham Road Farm Trails** has nearly 4 miles of trails that wind circuitously through open fields and managed forests. They were designed for cross-country skiing but are also open to pedestrian use in summer. The **Appalachian Trail** passes very close by and can be linked to via the Cossingham Trail. Southwest of I-91, the **Hazen Trail** runs 1.8 miles through woodlands above the Connecticut River.

Just across the Connecticut River in New Hampshire, the **Storrs Pond Recreation Area** in Hanover also features an extensive network of trails.

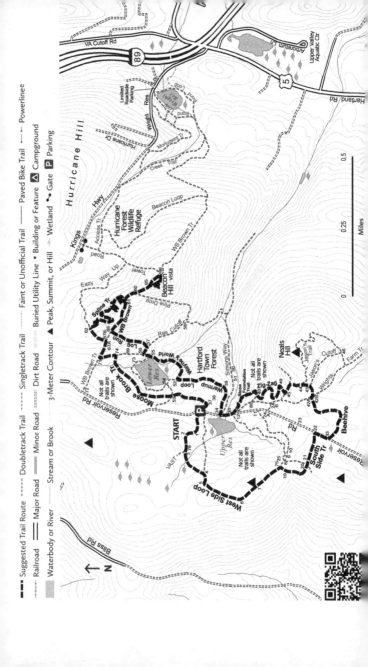

Legend:
- ▪▪ Suggested Trail Route
- ----- Doubletrack Trail
- ····· Faint or Unofficial Trail
- —— Paved Bike Trail
- ┴─┴ Powerline
- ····· Singletrack Trail
- ═══ Dirt Road
- ░░░ Buried Utility Line
- ■ Building or Feature
- ▲ Campground
- ┼┼┼ Railroad
- ═══ Minor Road
- ⟋⟋ 3-Meter Contour
- ▲ Peak, Summit, or Hill
- **P** Parking
- ═══ Major Road
- ---- Stream or Brook
- ⟋⟋ Wetland
- ⟍ Gate
- **P** Parking
- ≈≈ Waterbody or River

N ←

Miles: 0   0.25   0.5

Hurricane Hill

VA Cutoff Rd
89
5
Harland Rd
Upper Valley Aquatic Ctr
Arboretum Ln

Limited Roadside Parking
Wright Res
Pond Loop
Humlane Dr
Montgomery Tr
Creek Trail
Beacon Loop
Kings Hwy
Hurricane Forest Wildlife Refuge
Access Tr
WB Brown Tr
Eazy Way Up
Tower
Pine Drop
Beacon Hill vista
Spine Tr
WB Brown Tr
Res Cutoff
Log
Lower Res
Narnia
World
Moose Brook Tr
Not all trails are shown
Reservoir Rd
WB Brown Tr
Hartford Town Forest
Warmup Loop
Simons Way
Zig Zag
Foundations Trail
Not all trails are shown
Neals Hill
Jason's Trail
Jason's Cutoff
Wrights Cutoff
Farm Tr
START
P
VAST
Upper Res
P
Beehive
South Side Tr
Reservoir
West Side Loop
Not all trails are shown
Bliss Rd

DISTANCE 4 Miles **TOWN** Hartford

DIFFICULTY RATING Moderate **TRAIL STYLE** Loop

TRAIL TYPE Singletrack/Doubletrack **TOTAL ASCENT** 420 Feet

Hartford Town Forest (423 acres) and adjacent Hurricane Forest Wildlife Refuge (142 acres), sometimes collectively just called Hurricane Town Forest, contain a collection of hills between Quechee and White River Junction just west up the hill from the intersection of I-91 and I-89. A system of over ten miles of multi-use roads and trails of varying widths and difficulty levels surrounds a pair of former reservoirs (now wetlands) and connects the two properties. The suggested loop described here stays almost entirely on rolling hills within the town forest portion. See the optional extensions section for more. There are many junctions and intersections, so for legibility distances are noted for named full trail sections in the description rather than between each junction. All official intersections are numbered, and maps are posted at some intersections. Note that Hurricane Hill itself is actually off-property north of the trail system. Dogs are permitted off-leash in the town forest but must be under control, and must be leashed in the wildlife refuge.

DIRECTIONS   From I-89 Exit 1, take Rte. 4 east for 0.7 miles. Take a sharp right on Center of Town Road and go 0.7 miles uphill. Turn left onto Kings Highway and go 0.7 miles. Turn right on Reservoir Road and go 0.7 miles to the end.
GPS: "Hartford Town Forest, 683 Reservoir Rd"

TRAIL   From the parking area, look for a trailhead leading west, marked with yellow blazes. This is the start of West Side Loop, a wide doubletrack trail. Go west up to a junction (1), then bear right and briefly climb to another junction (2) where a VAST snowmobile corridor comes in on the right. Bear left and go up the hill to jct. 76 and jct. 3. Take a left and go southwest to jct. 4. Bear right and go slightly uphill to jct. 5 near the crest of the ridge. Go southwest to jct. 6, bear left and traverse the ridge over to jct. 7, then drop down to jct. 75. Total distance on West Side Trail is 0.7 miles.

Take a right and go south on South Slope Trail, immediately bearing left at jct. 19 and then staying straight at jct. 20 and jct. 21. Head east across the slope, passing a vernal pool on the right, to jct. 22. Total distance on South Slope Trail is 0.25 miles.

Go right on a class IV section of Reservoir Road and follow it 0.1 mile south. Go left on Beehive, a narrow singletrack trail. Follow it for 0.3 miles to jct. 42A, take a right and then an immediate left at 42B. Take the Zig-Zag Trail north, passing jct. 43 and jct. 44 on the right. From these two junctions, you can make a fun, somewhat challenging 0.6-mile extension that climbs around, up, and over 1,303-ft. Neals Hill. Descend Zig-Zag Trail to jct. 45 and take a right, then descend to jct. 49 and take a left, then descend to jct. 40 and go straight. Total distance on Zig-Zag Trail is about 0.6 miles.

Take a right at jct. 40 and follow Stone Foundation Trail down and around the slope for 0.1 mile to jct. 35 along Reservoir Road. Go right and head north a short distance, staying straight at jct. 35 and passing the Upper Reservoir wetland on your left, then go right at jct. 34.

Follow Warm-Up Loop east to jct. 36. Bear right and go east to jct. 39. Go straight and cross the slope heading north to jct. 52. Total distance on Warm-Up Trail is about 0.4 miles. Take a right and descend on Wayne's World, cross a creek below lower Reservoir, and climb to jct. 55. Go straight to jct. 56. Total distance on Wayne's World is about 0.3 miles. Take a right and go a short distance to jct. 57. Take a left and climb 0.1 mile up Log Run to jct. 68.

Go right and follow the wide W.B. Brown Trail east at a gentle grade up to an open field at the top of a 1,271-ft. hill, passing junctions 61, 60, and 65 along the way. Make a little loop around the tower, then come back west on W.B. Brown Trail. At jct. 61, go right on the swoopy singletrack of Spline Trail and follow it 0.4 miles up, down, and around the slope top jct. 62.

Take a left on Eazy Way Up and go 0.1 mile to jct. 67B. Take a right on W.B. Brown Trail and then immediately go straight at 67A. Descend 0.1 mile to a creek at jct. 71. Here, go left on the wide, purple-blazed Moose Brook Trail and follow it 0.5 miles south back to the trailhead, staying on it at junctions 70, 74, 53, and 37.

Optional Extensions The pedestrian-only trails are more challenging in steep-sloped Hurricane Forest to the east, which drops east down the hillside toward Rte. 5, but they are a great way to add on extra mileage and elevation (i.e., "vert"). Check out Beacon Loop, Pond Loop, Creek Trail, Monument Trail, and Access Trail. Limited parking is available at a trailhead by Wright Reservoir at the bottom.

NEARBY Just across the Connecticut River in New Hampshire, the **Boston Lot** in West Lebanon features a great network of trails, and **Farnum Hill Reserve** in Lebanon has seven miles of official trails accessible from five different trailheads.

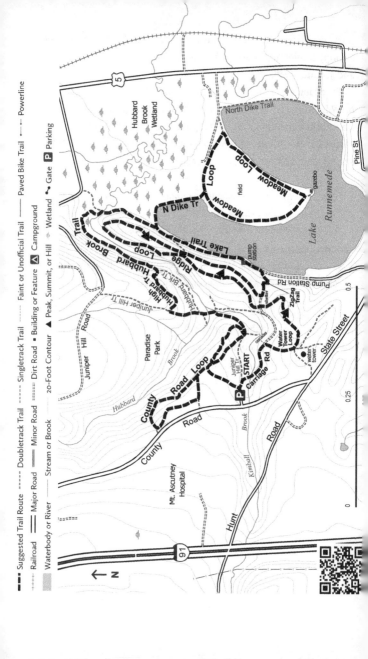

Legend:

■ ■ Suggested Trail Route - - - - Doubletrack Trail ------ Singletrack Trail ----- Faint or Unofficial Trail ——— Paved Bike Trail -+- Powerline

+++ Railroad ——— Major Road ====== Minor Road :::::: Dirt Road ▲ Peak, Summit, or Hill ⚑ Building or Feature △ Campground

——— Waterbody or River ——— Stream or Brook ——— 20-Foot Contour ▲ Peak, Summit, or Hill ⚑ Wetland ⚲ Gate P Parking

← N

Hubbard Brook Wetland

North Dike Trail

Meadow Loop

Meadow Loop

N Dike Tr

N Dike Tr Loop

Ridge Loop

Lake Trail

High Tr

Hubbard Brook Trail

Hubbard Brk Tr

Juniper Hill Road

Paradise Park

Hubbard Brook

Juniper Hill Tr

pump station

ZigZag Trail

Pump Station Rd

Lake Runnemede

gazebo

field

Pine St

Water Tower Loop

water tower

START

Juniper Hill Tr

Carriage Rd

Road Loop

County

County Road

Hubbard Brook

Kimball Brook

Mt. Ascutney Hospital

State Street

Road

Hunt Road

5

91

0   0.25   0.5

DISTANCE 4 Miles   **TOWN** Windsor
DIFFICULTY RATING Moderate   **TRAIL STYLE** Loop
TRAIL TYPE Singletrack   **TOTAL ASCENT** 325 Feet

Paradise Park in Windsor features a diverse network of signed but unmarked/unblazed trails. On the west side, the landscape consists of a series of steeply sloped forested ridges and eskers; the eastern half is mostly flat, with trails flanking Lake Runnemede and an active agricultural meadow. Some low-lying portions on the east side can be muddy, soggy, or even flooded in the spring, especially along the Meadow Loop and North Dike trails. Using many of the trails present, this loopy suggested route samples all of the site's terrain types. Though there are occasional rooty parts, trail surfaces are generally smooth and rock-free. Dogs are welcome but must be leashed. Swimming is not allowed in the lake.

DIRECTIONS From Rte. 5 in Windsor, take State Street 0.7 miles west. Veer right onto County Road and go 0.2 miles north to the parking area at the start of Paradise Park Road on the right.
GPS: "Paradise Park Parking Area"

TRAIL From the metal gate at the trailhead, go east on the wide dirt road. In a few hundred feet, bear right on Carriage Road and cross Kimball Brook on a small bridge. In 0.1 mile, take a right and climb briefly up the hill on the narrower Water Tower Loop trail. At the top, bear left at a fork and follow the trail across and down the hill to an open field.

   The next portion of the route features three parallel paths along a ridge. Go across the field and find the left branch of Ridge Trail, marked with a sign. Follow Ridge Trail 0.2 miles to a junction. Bear left and go 0.2 miles up to a tight curve to the right on a steep bluff at the north end of the ridge above Hubbard Brook. Go south on the parallel branch of Ridge Trail for 0.2 miles to a junction. Go straight and follow a level stretch of Ridge Trail 0.2 miles back to the field. A shelter lies ahead on the other side.

Bear left and find the start of Zig Zag Trail at the eastern end of the field. Take Zig Zag 0.1 mile down steep switchbacks to Lakeside Trail. Along a rugged narrow path, go north along the west short of Lake Runnemede for 0.25 miles to a junction. Go straight and drop 0.1 mile to a junction.

Starting a lollipop loop through the flat meadow and wetlands section, take a right on North Dike Trail and cross a stretch of boardwalks across a wet area. Curve right and go south along the grassy edge of the lake and up to a junction. In either direction, follow Meadow Loop for 0.8 miles in a ring around a farm field. There is a gazebo at the edge of the lake on the far side. Return via North Dike Trail to the junction with Lakeside Trail. Total lollipop loop distance is about a mile.

Go right and follow McLane Trail north along the bottom of the bluff to the left for 0.2 miles. Cross Hubbard Brook on a wooden bridge and then immediately bear left onto Hubbard Brook Trail at a junction. Follow the north side of the brook, curving left and heading southwest up into the narrow stream valley. In 0.2 miles, take a right and climb High Hubbard Trail up the hill. At a junction with Juniper Hill Trail, go left and descend 0.1 mile, passing a junction with Hubbard Brook Trail on the left and unmarked spur paths on the right.

Cross Hubbard Brook on a bridge, immediately pass a junction with a trail leading left across another bridge, then go 0.2 miles up the hill above a stream down to the left. At a fork just past a short spur on the left leading down to a small waterfall over some ledges in the stream, bear right onto County Road Loop.

Go northwest up the hill on the east side of County Road Loop for 0.4 miles, passing multiple paths and connector links leading left along the way. Near the upper end, curve left and then drop down the west side of the loop for 0.2 miles back to the trailhead, staying right at all junctions (except one spur leading a short distance out to the road).

NEARBY The many trails of **Mount Ascutney** lie just a few miles southwest (see next two sites). Just across the Connecticut River in New Hampshire, **Saint-Gaudens National Historical Park** in Plainfield features a small but diverse network of nature trails.

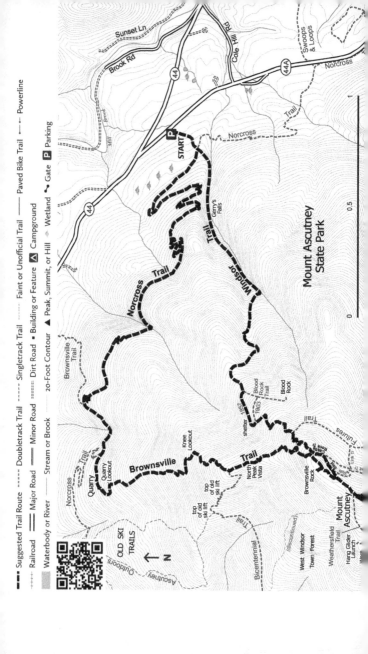

Legend (top):

Suggested Trail Route ···· Doubletrack Trail ----- Singletrack Trail ----- Faint or Unofficial Trail — Paved Bike Trail ⤍ Powerline

+++ Railroad — Major Road ═══ Minor Road ⋯⋯ Dirt Road ▪ Building or Feature Ⓐ Campground

— Waterbody or River — Stream or Brook ──── 20-Foot Contour ▲ Peak, Summit, or Hill ☀ Wetland • Gate 🅿 Parking

Sunset Ln

Brook Rd

Cole Hill Rd

44

44A

Norcross

Swoops & Loops

Mill

🅿 START

Norcross

Trail

Norcross

Mount Ascutney State Park

Gerry's Falls

Windsor Trail

Norcross Trail

0.5

1

0

Brownsville Trail

Quarry Trail

Norcross Trail

Quarry Lookout

Knee Lookout

Brownsville Trail

top of old ski lift

top of old ski lift

Trail

North Peak Vista

Brownsville Rock

shelter

Blood Rock Trail

Blood Rock

Futures

Trail

Rock Tr

Slalom Tr

Trail

Bicentennial

OLD SKI TRAILS

← N

Mount Ascutney

West Windsor Town Forest

Weathersfield Trail

Hang Glider Launch

(discontinued)

Ascutney Outdoors

DISTANCE 7.5 Miles   **TOWN** Windsor and West Windsor
DIFFICULTY RATING Challenging   **TRAIL STYLE** Loop
TRAIL TYPE Singletrack   **TOTAL ASCENT** 2,526 Feet

Born of ancient volcanic forces, Mount Ascutney towers over the surrounding landscape, a monadnock peak looming high over the rolling hills of the Connecticut River Valley. Four main hiking trails (Windsor, Brownsville, Weathersfield, and Futures) climb through Mount Ascutney State Park to the prominent 3,130-ft. summit, as does a paved auto road. A less-frequently used fifth trail (Bicentennial Trail) ascends through the Ascutney Trails network on the mountain's west side. All trail routes are rugged and challenging, but each has excellent scenic vistas and unique geologic features. Semi-hidden gems to visit include old quarries, trailside waterfalls, a hang-glider launching spot, granite outcrops, and a "Steam Donkey" (old logging machinery). This suggested route combines two of the main trails and a connector trail to form a challenging, medium-length loop, though many different combinations and variations are possible and worthwhile. In the park, which covers the summit and most of the northeast side of the mountain, bikes are only permitted on designated trails such as Norcross Trail and Swoops and Loops. Dogs are allowed but must be leashed at all times. Note that these trails are very popular and parking lots often fill up, especially on weekends.

DIRECTIONS From I-91 Exit 7, take Rte. 12 down to Rte. 5, then go north for 1.2 miles. Carefully bear left at a fork onto Rte. 44A/Back Mountain Road and go 2.8 miles northwest up the hill, under the highway, and past the main state park entrance to the Windsor Trail parking lot on the left.

TRAIL   From the trailhead, take the white-blazed Windsor Trail south up the grassy hill for 0.15 miles to the edge of the woods. In a few hundred more feet, go straight at an intersection with Norcross Trail. Climb 0.5 miles southwest at an increasingly steeper grade above a brook to a junction with a short spur path leading left down to Gerry's Falls.

From the spur path, continue climbing at a steep, steady grade. Cross several brooks, then bear right and climb northwest away from the stream valley. At 1.5 miles, go right on Windsor Trail/1867 Trail at a junction with a steep blue-blazed trail leading left up to Blood Rock, a small ledge above a very steep drop-off. Climb up to a log shelter and spring on the right, then curve left and arrive at a junction with an upper trail (1903 Route) leading left towards Blood Rock at 1.75 miles. This way to Blood Rock is a little easier, but both options involve some steep climbing and descending.

Climb steeply for 0.3 miles up switchbacks into spruce-fir forest. At a junction with Futures Trail on the left, go right and climb another 0.2 miles at a slightly gentler grade to a junction in a level area. Go left a few hundred feet on blue-blazed Castle Rock Trail across a mossy, bouldery area to a spur leading left to Castle Rock, where there is a great east-facing vista. Go a short distance further south to a junction. Bear right on Slot Trail and go 0.1 mile southwest across the slope to a junction. Bear right on Slab Trail, pass a junction with Windsor Trail, and gently climb 0.2 miles west to the observation tower. The actual summit is 0.1 mile further west.

Backtrack to the start of Windsor Trail and follow it 0.1 mile northeast across the ridge to Ascutney North, where a side trail drops 0.1 mile left over to Brownsville Rock, which has an expansive west-facing vista. From Ascutney North, go 0.1 mile further northeast to a junction.

Take a left and descend the white-blazed Brownsville Trail, sometimes gently and sometimes very steeply (see figure 10). On the way down, pass the view ledges of North Peak Vista at 0.5 miles, a junction with the newly re-routed Bicentennial Trail on the left at 0.7 miles, Knee Lookout at 0.9 miles, and Quarry Lookout at 1.6 miles. The trail can be a bit tough on the feet in places along this stretch, with innumerable sharp rocks and trip-hazard tree roots, so caution is warranted. After dropping down a steep ledge face on stone steps, the trail reaches the open rocky rubble pile (grout) of Norcross Quarry at 1.8 miles, where there are remnants of the old granite mining operation and an open western view. At 1.9 miles, pass a junction with Norcross Trail leading down to Ascutney Trails. Continue descending on Brownsville Trail, now at a gentler grade on a wide old road heading east, to a fork at 2.2 miles.

Bear right and take the blue-blazed, singletrack Norcross Trail 2.8 miles southeast across the steep-sided lower slopes of the mountain back to Windsor Trail. There are several long switchbacks in this section, as well as a few wooden bridges over steep stream drainages, boardwalks over wet areas, and a couple of rough, rocky spots, but all of it is at an easy grade and it's easy to follow (no junctions or intersections). Back at Windsor Trail, go left and descend to return to the trailhead.

Optional Extension   A somewhat similar but nearly twice as long loop can be made by swapping out the steep Windsor Trail with the 4.8-mile Futures Trail to the south. This option requires a longer traverse on (a mostly easier section of) Norcross Trail, but offers a more gradual ascent of the mountain on Futures (though the first mile is still pretty steep).

NEARBY From the main state park entrance about 1.5 miles southeast, the **Futures Trail** offers the longest climb up the mountain, though it is still rugged and challenging. Across the street from the park entrance station, the new **Swoops and Loops** trail does just what it suggests in the woods below Rte. 44A; it was built specifically as a mountain-bike trail and they have priority on it, but it's also open to pedestrian use (just be extra alert for and always yield to other users).

Just across the Connecticut River in New Hampshire, **Cornish Town Forest** features a network of trails on the south side of Wellmans Hill, as does **Moody Park** in Claremont.

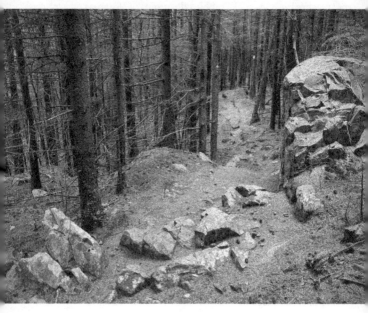

FIGURE 10. Brownsville Trail near the top of Mount Ascutney in Windsor.

DISTANCE 3.9 Miles   **TOWN** West Windsor and Windsor

DIFFICULTY RATING Moderate   **TRAIL STYLE** Loop

TRAIL TYPE Singletrack   **TOTAL ASCENT** 470 Feet

The lower northwest slopes of Mount Ascutney feature an extensive trail system called Ascutney Trails. Formerly known as Ascutney Basin, this spectacular network may be accessed from trailheads at the base of the former ski area as well as a parking area at West Windsor Town Forest. The trails are managed by Ascutney Trails Association (ATA) with the mission of "supporting human-powered recreation in the Mt. Ascutney area." This short, suggested route samples some of the site's most "runnable" highlights but represents just a fraction of the options available. On the north side of the mountain, the well-built and well-graded Norcross Trail connects this network to the hiking trails of Mount Ascutney State Park to the northeast. The recently re-routed Bicentennial Trail climbs up the west side to the upper end of the new Ascutney Outdoors Trail at the top of the old ski trails, and to the upper part of the Brownsville Trail near the top of the ridge.

DIRECTIONS   From I-91 Exit 7, take Rte. 12 down to Rte. 5, then go north for 1.2 miles. Carefully bear left at a fork onto Rte. 44A and go 3 miles northwest. Bear left onto Rte. 44 and go 2 miles west. Turn left on Ski Tow Road and go 0.5 miles up to the Ascutney Outdoors Center's large dirt parking lot on the right.

A smaller alternate trailhead for the Ascutney Trails system can be found just southwest of Mile-Long Field at the West Windsor Town Forest trailhead on Coaching Lane.

GPS: "Ascutney Outdoors Ski Tow Road"

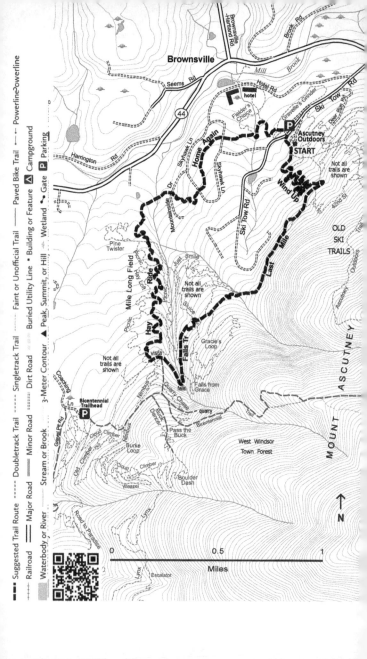

Legend

- ▪▪ Suggested Trail Route
- +++ Railroad
- ~~~ Waterbody or River
- ----- Doubletrack Trail
- ═══ Minor Road
- ⋯⋯ 3-Meter Contour
- ⋯⋯ Faint or Unofficial Trail
- ═══ Major Road
- ▲ Peak, Summit, or Hill
- ----- Singletrack Trail
- ⋯⋯ Dirt Road
- ~~~ Stream or Brook
- ——— Paved Bike Trail
- ⋯⋯ Buried Utility Line
- ✦ Wetland
- +—+ Powerline
- • Building or Feature
- ⌐ Gate
- 🅿 Parking
- 🅰 Campground

Brownsville

hotel

Ascutney Outdoors
START

44

Seems Rd
Hotel Rd
Gravele's Grinder
Ski Tow Rd
Brownsville-Hartland Rd
Brook Rd
Deer Rd

Harrington Rd
Skyhawk Ln
Home Again
Fielder's Choice
Skyhawk Ln
Wind Up
Not all trails are shown
42nd St

Mountainside Dr
Pine Twister
Just Smile
Last Mile
OLD SKI TRAILS

Mile Long Field
Ride
Picnic
Slice
Ascutney Outdoors
Ascutney

Hay
Falls Tr
Gracie's Loop
MOUNT ASCUTNEY

vista
Nimbus
Quarry Chase
falls
Falls from Grace

Coasting
Cloud Ln
Bicentennial Trailhead 🅿
Cloud Climber
Old Climber
Nimbus
Pass the Buck
Burke Loop
quarry
Bicentennial Trail

Gravel Pit Rd
Cloud Climber
Weazel
Boulder Dash
West Windsor Town Forest

Road to Paradise
Lynx
Lynx
Escalator

0   0.5   1
Miles

↑ N

TRAIL From the parking lot, follow the dirt driveway up the hill to the Ascutney Outdoors Center (AOC). Find the trailhead to the right of the building, and follow Last Mile trail southwest up the grassy slope. Just past a small building with a deck, curve left to a junction. Go right and ascend the Wind Up trail as it climbs at a gentle grade for 0.5 miles up the lower slope of the mountain via a series of tight switchback wiggles along an old ski trail and its adjacent wooded margins. The trail construction is truly impressive here.

At a junction, bear right back onto Last Mile and go southwest across the slope at a nearly level grade for about 0.6 miles. The trail braids several times, with preferred directionality clearly marked with arrows. From a junction where Just Smile and Utility Road lead down to the right, continue southwest down the slope at a gentle grade for 0.4 miles on Last Mile, passing multiple junctions on either side.

> *Optional Extension* Just upslope from the southern half of Last Mile, Gracie's Loop makes a nearly mile-long circuit up, across, and down the hillside. It connects with Last Mile at two close intersections.

From an intersection with Sluice and Deer Run trails, go left to follow the southernmost part of Last Mile for 0.2 miles to an intersection with Raina's Run down to the right and Falls from Grace trail above on the left. Go straight on Falls Trail and follow it for 0.25 miles as it leads down into a ravine with a waterfall, crosses in front of the falls on a boardwalk bridge, and climbs out the other side of the stream valley.

At a junction with Cort's Jester trail leading right, Falls Trail emerges into the open at the upper, southeast corner of a large, north-sloping hayfield called Mile-Long Field. Go about a hundred feet out into the field to a picnic table near a junction with the lower end of Nimbus trail on the left.

> *Optional Extension* Upslope from Mile-Long Field, a fun but navigationally complicated lollipop loop can be made using Nimbus, Cloud Climber, and Pass the Buck trails. Total extra distance is around 3 miles

but it is significantly more challenging and there are many confusing junctions along the way; it pays to learn the network by going further and further with successive visits and figuring it out in stages.

Starting about a third of the way across the top of Mile-Long Field, take Hay Ride trail down through the scenic meadow. Finding the start may be tricky at certain times of the year, but you'll see it soon enough. The trail descends for nearly a mile via a flowing series of curves on the right/east side of the field, occasionally skimming the woods and passing junctions with Cort's Jester trail. This is about as close to cross-country running as it gets, friends. At the bottom of the hill, take a right on Picnic trail, which soon becomes a grassy dirt road, and follow it northeast for 0.2 miles to Mountainside Drive.

Cross the road and enter the woods on Home Again trail. Climb 0.2 miles up the hillside at a gentle grade, via a series of switchbacks, to Skyhawk Lane. With permission, this section passes through a private residential neighborhood and quiet is requested by the residents. Descend slightly for 0.3 miles, passing several homes along the way, to another intersection with Skyhawk Lane. Cross the road and follow Home Again for 0.3 miles down and up across the slope back to the parking lot, passing several junctions with trails on the left leading down to resort buildings.

NEARBY From the **West Windsor Town Forest** trailhead in the southern half of the Ascutney Trails network, several notably fun trails to run are Lynx, Nirvana, Southern Belle, Ridgeback, Rock & Roll, Grassy Knoll, and South Ridge Run. On the north side of the mountain, the new **Norcross Trail** links the Ascutney Trails system with **Mount Ascutney State Park** trails. Several relatively nearby mid-size mountains like Little Ascutney Mountain in Weathersfield and Hawks Mountain in Cavendish have rough routes to their summits, but they're neither marked nor maintained as hiking trails.

DISTANCE 4.8 Miles   **TOWN** Springfield and Weathersfield
DIFFICULTY RATING Moderate   **TRAIL STYLE** Out-and-Back
TRAIL TYPE Doubletrack/Singletrack   **TOTAL ASCENT** 423 Feet

North Springfield Reservoir is a U.S. Army Corps of Engineers (ACOE) flood control area flanking portions of Black River and North Branch Black River upstream of the 120-ft. high, 610-ft. wide North Springfield Dam. A variety of trail types line the east side of the river valley, ranging from wide dirt roads to narrow singletrack hiking trails. The terrain is gently rolling with occasional steep pitches and flat sections. This suggested route follows a north–south path from Sand Hill Trail in the north to a trail network at the Eleanor Ellis Springweather Nature Area further south. The trails are not particularly well signed or marked, but they are fairly easy to follow. For a longer option, an 8.4-mile loop can be made all the way around the reservoir, but it requires following 1.3 miles of paved road in Perkinsville on the northwest side. Note that low portions may be flooded (by design) or muddy in spring and early summer or after heavy rains.

DIRECTIONS   From Springfield, take Rte. 106 northwest for 2.4 miles. Bear right on Reservoir Road and go 4.1 miles north. At a curve to the left this becomes Stoughton Pond Road. Go west 0.2 miles. The trailhead parking area, also known as Fisherman's Parking, is on the left just before the dam.
GPS: "Sand Hill Trail Stoughton Pond Road"

TRAIL   From the big brown sign by the parking area, follow the mowed path south a few hundred feet across a field to a metal gate at the edge of the woods. This is the start of Sand Hill Trail, though it isn't marked as such anywhere on-site. Drop steeply down a gravel

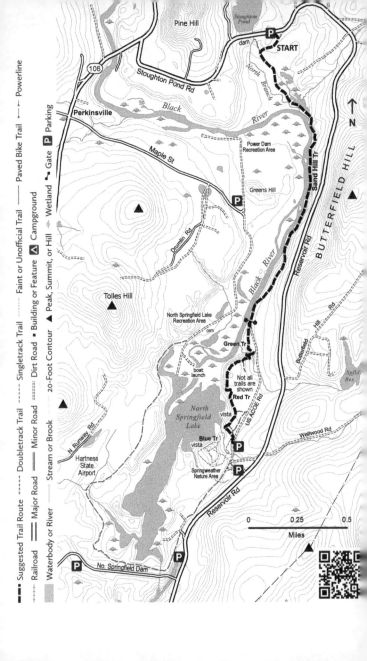

Suggested Trail Route · · · · Doubletrack Trail · · · · Singletrack Trail · · · · · Faint or Unofficial Trail · · · · Paved Bike Trail ←→ Powerline
+++ Railroad ═══ Major Road ══ Minor Road ═══ Dirt Road ▪ Building or Feature ▲ Campground
▬ Waterbody or River ∿ Stream or Brook ⌇ 20-Foot Contour ▲ Peak, Summit, or Hill ⬥ Wetland ● Gate 🅿 Parking

Stoughton Pond

Pine Hill

🅿

dam

START

106

Stoughton Pond Rd

North Branch

Perkinsville

Black

River

Power Dam
Recreation Area

Maple St

🅿

Greens Hill

BUTTERFIELD HILL

Sand Hill Tr

Drumlin Rd

Reservoir Rd

Black River

Tolles Hill

North Springfield Lake
Recreation Area

cem

Green Tr

Butterfield

Hill
Rd

Spfld
Res

boat
launch

Not all
trails are
shown

Red Tr

US ACOE Rd

vista

N. Runway Rd

North
Springfield
Lake

Blue Tr

vista

🅿

Wellwood Rd

Hartness
State
Airport

🅿

Springweather
Nature Area

▲

Reservoir Rd

0   0.25   0.5

Miles

🅿

🅿

No. Springfield Dam

▲

path to a junction with a dirt road and bear right, heading toward the river. The road emerges from the woods and becomes grassy. At a junction where a path leads right up toward the Stoughton Pond dam, go left.

Follow the wide, mown path south along a raised berm between open wetland marshes just east of North Branch Black River. At 0.5 miles the trail enters the woods near the confluence of Black River and North Branch at the south end of the marshes. For the next 1.1 miles the wide trail undulates up and down multiple times on a woods road along the lower western slopes of Butterfield Hill, passing numerous scenic views out across the river (and the unfortunate blight of dense invasive shrubs choking the floodplain terrace on the other side). Sand Hill Trail ends at a gate just before a paved turnaround bulb at the lower end of an ACOE service road.

Cross the end of the circular bulb and look for the trail on the other side. This is the north end of Green Trail, one of three color-blazed, "self-guided" trail loops of the Eleanor Ellis Springweather Nature Area. Bikes are not allowed on the trails south of this point. A mown path passes through some shrubs, crosses a wooden bridge, rises through a field, and then curves left and becomes a small dirt road. Just before reaching the service road, turn right at a green-blazed wooden post. Continuing south on the now narrow Green Trail, descend to a stream crossing, then rise along a switchback up a steeply sloped hillside.

At a junction near the top of the bluff, the Green Trail meets the Red Trail loop, which can be followed via either branch. For now, go right and pass through pine forest along the edge of the bluff above the river. The trail emerges at a flat meadow with benches and picnic tables called The Gathering Place overlooking the north end of North Springfield Lake. At the other end of the field, follow Red Trail into the woods. The intersections get a little confusing here. Stay right at two junctions, following Red Trail around the bluff and then down the slope to a junction with Blue Trail where there is a wooden bench above a small stream. A short wood-railing-lined path leads left up to the East Access/Springweather trailhead from here. Return back to the northern trailhead the way you came, or continue south for the full 8.4-mile loop around the reservoir.

NEARBY Just south of the turnaround, the Blue Trail singletrack path continues south through the woods, crossing a stream on a wooden bridge and then rising gently to a lightly maintained warren of narrow paths marked with blue-blazed posts; exploring this network adds roughly one extra mile to the suggested route. North of Stoughton Pond Road, **Branch Brook Trail** partially encircles Stoughton Pond, though some paved road is required to complete the southern half of the loop, including a stretch across the top of the dam. There is a designated swimming area on the west side of Stoughton Pond.

DISTANCE 4.9 Miles (3.7 at Muckross; 1.2 in Hartness)   **TOWN** Springfield

DIFFICULTY RATING Moderate   **TRAIL STYLE** Out-and-Back

TRAIL TYPE Doubletrack/Singletrack   **TOTAL ASCENT** 550 Feet (435 Feet at Muckross; 115 Feet in Hartness

When combined, the small trail systems at Muckross State Park and Hartness Park in Springfield Town Forest make a nice, uncrowded trail-run option if you are in the Springfield area or looking for something a little different. The suggested route combines trails at both sites. Located on the grounds of a former estate, Muckross is named after a building in Ireland's Killarney National Park. It is a new park, currently still undeveloped, that includes numerous old lodges, cabins, and cottages; a trout pond; and roads on the site. Hartness Park includes the now-overgrown track of a former ski jump; trails are blazed with colored rectangles, and key trail junctions and features are marked with numbered posts. Both sites lie along a long north–south ridge of hills extending south from 1,545-ft. Camp Hill about four miles north.

DIRECTIONS From Exit 7 off of I-91, take Rte. 11 northwest for 1 mile. Turn right on Paddock Road, cross the Toonerville Trail bike path and the bridge over Black River, then turn left on Muckross Road and go 400 feet up the hill. The small parking area just inside the park fits about 6 vehicles. When it's full, alternate parking can be found one or two miles southeast at the Toonerville Trail trailhead or the Exit 7 Park & Ride.

There is no official parking area for Hartness Park at the north end, though it can be accessed from a cul-de-sac at the end of Dell Road below and to the west.

GPS: "26 Muckross Road"

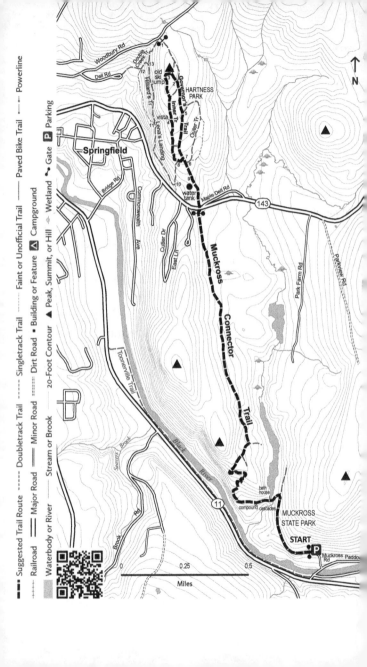

Legend (top):

- : Suggested Trail Route
- ---- Doubletrack Trail
- ----- Singletrack Trail
- ······· Faint or Unofficial Trail
- ---- Paved Bike Trail
- -·-·- Powerline
- ++++ Railroad
- ═══ Major Road
- ═══ Minor Road
- ::::::: Dirt Road
- • Building or Feature
- ▲ Campground
- —— Stream or Brook
- —— Waterbody or River
- —— 20-Foot Contour
- ▲ Peak, Summit, or Hill
- ✦ Wetland
- ◆ Gate
- P Parking

Map labels:

Woodbury Rd

Dell Rd

Doane's Creek

13
12

old ski jump

Hillard's Tr.

Governor's Inner Trail

HARTNESS PARK

vista

Lena's Landing

Outer Tr.

5
6 7
8

Springfield

Bridge Rd

Commonwealth Ave

Cutler Dr

East Ln

water tank

10
9

Maple Dell Rd

143

Muckross Connector Trail

Park Farm Rd

Parkview Rd

Toonerville Trail

Black River

Sawyers Brook

Brook Rd

11

bath house

compound cascades

MUCKROSS STATE PARK

START P

Muckross Paddock Rd

N ↑

0   0.25   0.5

Miles

TRAIL   From the parking area, go west through a gate and follow the dirt road west and then north up the hill, staying on the road at several junctions with smaller side roads. At the top of the rise, curve left and follow the road down the hill and over a bridge (a faint path here leads left down to a ledgy waterfall), past a spur road leading right over to the dam and pond, and down to a compound of old buildings in a field.

Staying on the right side of the compound, look for the start of Muckross Connector Trail at the edge of the woods just past a garage on the left and small shed on the right. The trail is marked with yellow-diamond signs with black arrows. Follow Muckross Connector northwest for 0.4 miles, climbing the hill at a gentle grade via switchbacks. Cross over the crest of the ridge and pass a spur trail on the right, then descend 0.1 mile to a junction.

Bear left and follow the trail north up the slope for 0.4 miles. Along this stretch the trail leaves the park and enters private property. It soon levels off and traverses the side of the ridge for 0.5 miles through a recently harvested woodland with a grassy understory; parts of the trail may be soggy here. At an old road along the south boundary of a campground, bear slightly left and climb 0.2 miles up the hill.

Cross over Rte. 143, then enter Hartness Park on the other side, just to the left of Maple Dell Road. Follow the wide road up the hill. Just past a water tank on the left, enter the woods on a doubletrack-width trail at jct. 9. Follow the trail north to jct. 6. Continue a few more feet to jct. 7, then take a left and follow Inner Trail north up the ridge for 0.3 miles, passing several trails leading right at unmarked junctions and a picnic table with a view out over Springfield at jct. 4.

Near the summit, a short spur path leads left down to the top of an overgrown old ski jump that dropped west down the steep slope towards town. Continuing over the top, bear right at jct. 3, then right again at an unmarked junction, then descend briefly to jct. 2. Follow Governor's Trail down the ridge back to jct. 6, passing jcts. 5 and 7 along the way and ignoring two unmarked connector paths leading to the right. Return south back to Muckross the way you came.

Optional Extensions   There are several other trails at Hartness Park to create small loops with. Two notable options include the short and easy, red-blazed Outer Loop path on the east side of the ridge, and the longer alternate routes of Hillard's Trail and Lena's Landing, which traverse the west side of the hill below the steep Double Creek Trail; the lower, western trails are significantly more challenging due to occasional steep pitches. There are also a few existing spur trails at Muckross, though they do not currently go all the way around the pond.

NEARBY A few miles south, there are several rough, unmarked trails to the top of 1,470-ft. **Mount Ephraim**. Across the Connecticut River in New Hampshire, there are fun trail networks at **Fall Mountain State Forest** in Langdon and **Mount Kilburn** in North Walpole.

DISTANCE 5.5 Miles   **TOWN** Athens and Grafton
DIFFICULTY RATING Moderate   **TRAIL STYLE** Out-and-Back
TRAIL TYPE Singletrack   **TOTAL ASCENT** 945 Feet

Athens Dome is a hilly area of geologic uplift just south of Saxtons River in the towns of Athens and Grafton where a broad "dome" of ancient rocks protrude up above the surrounding landscape. The northern end of the dome features a network of marked trails that visit a variety of the area's natural features, including huge boulders, scenic hilltop vistas, open and forested wetlands, tumbling brooks, and a centuries-old soapstone quarry. All trails are marked with colored yellow discs and there are signposts with mileages at key junctions and intersections. The trails were built and are maintained by the Windmill Hill Pinnacle Association (WHPA), who own much of the land, and Grafton Improvement Association. This suggested route incorporates many of the trails in the system. It is possible to link directly from here to the larger Windmill Ridge trail network to the east and south via the Sleepy Hollow Trail, and from there go all the way south to Putney Mountain (and soon beyond) on trails.

DIRECTIONS   From Bellows Falls, take Rte. 121 about 8 miles through Saxons River towards Grafton. Turn left on Ledge Road/Town Highway 83 and go 0.9 miles up to a parking area. The last quarter mile or so of the road can be rough and is not maintained in winter. GPS: "Athens Dome Trail"

TRAIL   From the parking area, look for the trailhead next to a map kiosk. Follow the curvy set of log steps up the hill, then ascend the white-blazed Creature Rock Trail up through mature hardwood forest. At about 0.2 miles you come to Creature Rock, a house-sized pile of

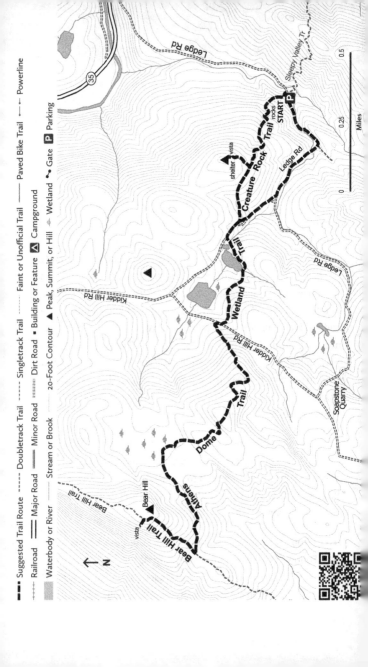

large boulders surrounded by scraggly trees. Bear right and continue following Creature Rock Trail west up to a junction.

Take a right and follow the yellow-blazed spur trail north up to 1,300-ft. Lake Summit where there is a camping shelter, and an east-facing vista overlooking Cambridgeport and Atcherson Hollow below. Then return south back to the junction, go right and follow Creature Rock Trail west across and down the slope to a junction.

Take a right and follow white-blazed Wetland Trail northwest up the hill for about 0.1 mile to a junction. Turn left and follow Wetland Trail west for 0.5 miles up the slope to a junction with Kidder Hill Road, passing a pair of open wetlands on the right along the way.

Cross the woods road onto Athens Dome Trail. Climb 0.5 miles at a steady grade to the top of a hill (presumably Athens Dome itself, though it isn't named that on maps). Drop down the other side of the hill and cross the slope for about 0.7 miles to a junction, passing a forested spruce wetland on the right along the way. Take a right and follow the blue-blazed Bear Hill Trail 0.25 miles up the ridge to the spruce-covered, 1,740-ft. summit of Bear Hill. There is a west-facing vista down a short spur trail near the top.

From Bear Hill, return back south on Bear Hill Trail and then east on Athens Dome Trail and Wetland Trails back to the intersection with Creature Rock Trail, a distance of 2.1 miles. Go straight and follow a linking trail 0.15 miles down the hill to a junction. Bear left and follow Ledge Road 0.6 miles east along Ledge Road Brook back down to the trailhead.

Optional Extensions

1. You can turn this route into a figure-8 loop of similar distance by continuing north along the ridge from Bear Hill. The half-mile, semi-technical descent over mossy, rocky ledges beneath spruce and hemlock trees is rip-roaring fun, then the trail briefly traverses right across the slope and reaches an old road. Bearing left, descend the rough road to a kiosk at a small parking area. Go right on Kidder Hill Road

and climb 1 mile southeast past the end of the maintained road to a junction. From there, bear left at a fork and follow a trail 0.4 miles southeast back to the Creature Rock Trail junction.

2. To extend the route by about a mile, head back down Bear Hill Trail and take Athens Dome Trail 1.1 miles east back to Kidder Hill Road as suggested above, but then go right on the road up and follow it 0.5 miles southwest up and over a rise to a junction. Take a left on Ledge Road and follow it east. In about 0.15 miles, pass the old Soapstone Quarry on the right (there is an information kiosk here). Continue east down Ledge Road for 1 mile to a junction, then bear right and follow the road 0.6 miles back to the trailhead.

3. On the other side of the parking lot, the mile-long Sleepy Valley Trail leads east to a trailhead along Rte. 35. After crossing a stream on a sturdy bridge, it climbs steeply for 0.5 miles to the crest of a ridge, then drops just as steeply down the other side, passing through a wooded boulder field about halfway down. Return back the way you came.

NEARBY Just west of Bear Hill, on the hillside below the summit, the **Grafton Trails & Outdoor Center** offers a system of cross-country ski, mountain bike, and hiking trails. To the southeast, **Windmill Ridge Nature Reserve** (owned by WHPA) and the **Putney Mountain Association** lands cohost an extensive system of lovely trails along the Windmill Ridge from Rockingham and Athens south to Putney. This network has multiple trailheads on both sides of the ridge, including the Sleepy Valley Trail parking area mentioned in the optional extension above.

About eight miles east, near the mouth of the Saxtons River just south of Bellows Falls, **Bald Mountain** (another WHPA property) features a dense network of relatively short trails. Though the peak itself is forested and sports only limited views, the site's overall variety is notable, with a broad mix of terrain types, trail widths, and difficulty levels; plus, there are ledges next to a cool but dangerous waterfall that can be reached with some steep scrambling.

DISTANCE 3.9 Miles   **TOWN** Westminster

DIFFICULTY RATING Moderate   **TRAIL STYLE** Lollipop Loop

TRAIL TYPE Singletrack   **TOTAL ASCENT** 645 Feet

The Windmill Ridgeline runs north–south between Saxtons River in the north and Newfane in the south. Crowning Windmill Ridge near its center is a 1,637-ft. peak called The Pinnacle, from which there is an excellent west-facing view. Along the ridge and an adjacent one to the west, a system of trails (with a few short road sections) connects Athens Dome in the north with Putney Mountain and adjacent properties to the south. The trail network is largely owned and managed by Windmill Hill Pinnacle Association (WHPA) and Putney Mountain Association. This suggested route follows a lollipop route that climbs up and over the peak from the east, combining sections of three primary trails and providing a tantalizing sampling of all the ridge has to offer. The entire route lies on Windmill Ridge Nature Reserve land, and coincides with the Walk Through Time Interpretive Trail. The trails are very well marked, easy to follow, and great for running; footing is generally excellent and grades are rarely steep. Various extensions are possible, and a long point-to-point trek along the ridge is highly recommended. Note that these trails are closed temporarily during mud season in early spring to prevent erosion to them, the parking area, and the access road.

DIRECTIONS From Putney, take Kimball Hill Road/Westminster Road north for 1.7 miles. At a junction, turn left and go 2.7 miles north on Hickory Ridge Road (stay straight at a fork where Tavern Hill Road leads left). At a junction, take a left on West Road and go 1.9 miles west and north. Turn left onto Windmill Hill Road North and go 1 mile west and south up the hill to the trailhead on the right. Note

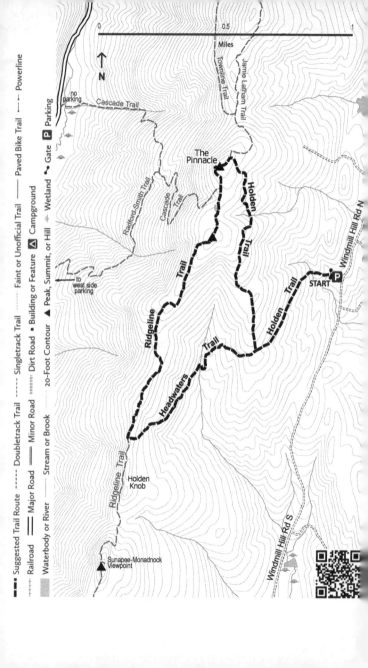

that the last mile of road is often closed to all but local traffic during Vermont's infamous mud season.

GPS: "Pinnacle Trailhead, Holden Trail; 1026 Windmill Hill Road North"

TRAIL   From the kiosk at the trailhead, go west past an ornate metal gate on the wide Holden Trail (an old road blazed with red discs). At about 0.2 miles, curve left just after crossing a small stream and begin ascending southwest at a gentle grade, occasionally rising over exposed bedrock outcrops. Near the crest of a sub-ridge at 0.5 miles, pass a junction where Holden Trail goes right and continue straight over the ridge and down the other side on Headwaters Trail (marked with blue discs). The trail gets narrower here and winds around the slope a bit more. In about 0.3 miles, just past a stone wall, descend to cross the headwaters trickle of Sacketts Brook and then climb at a moderate grade for 0.4 miles up to the crest of Windmill Ridge.

Optional Extension   Take a left at the junction and follow Ridgeline Trail 0.6 miles south along the crest of the ridge. You'll cross over Holden Knob and then climb a switchback up to an unnamed hill (1,152 feet) where there is an east-facing vista that includes Mount Sunapee and Mount Monadnock at a bench. Total round-trip distance to and from the vista is 1.2 miles.

Turn right and follow Ridgeline Trail 1.3 miles north to the top of The Pinnacle. This section is a highlight of any trip. Blazed with white discs, the trail undulates along the ridge, gradually rising as it goes. In a small saddle about a quarter of a mile from the summit, pass a small pond on the left and then a junction shortly afterwards where Cascade Trail descends toward Hedgehog Gulf on the left (the combined Radford-Smith and Cascade trails make an excellent two-mile-long approach from the west, utilizing many switchbacks and well-graded stretches). As the trail nears the top of the mountain, the forest understory fills with sedges beneath a canopy of oaks and hop hornbeam, creating a strikingly appealing savannah-like scene.

The trail soon emerges out into the open and reaches The Pinnacle, where there is a restored hiker's cabin and a terrific west-facing vista with rock benches. From the summit, go 0.1 mile north to a junction.

Optional Extension From the junction just north of The Pinnacle, go straight on Jamie Latham Trail. A rolling, 3-mile trek north along the ridge on this trail and the Hemlock Trail brings you to Paul's Ledges where there is a spectacular view from open bedrock outcrops in a small meadow.

Turn right and follow red-blazed Holden Trail for 0.9 miles southeast down the ridge. Back at the junction with Headwaters Trail, turn left and descend 0.5 miles back down to the trailhead.

NEARBY A bounty of often steep trails lead up to **Windmill Ridge** from either side. Notable ones in the immediate vicinity include Windmill Hill Trail (rough and steep), Parsons Cutoff (very lightly used), Ed Dodd Trail, Townline Trail, Cascade Trail, and Radford-Smith Trail. The latter two are closed during winter and reopen in mid-April. Some lack parking at the bottom; check current Windmill Hill Pinnacle Association maps online for updates. Of the other side trails listed, Radford-Smith Trail and Townline Trail are the best for running. Near Paul's Ledges, the Undercliff Trail, Hemlock Trail, and Sugar Grove Trail are all also great for running.

DISTANCE 5.3 Miles   **TOWN** Brookline and Putney
DIFFICULTY RATING Moderate   **TRAIL STYLE** Loop
TRAIL TYPE Singletrack   **TOTAL ASCENT** 860 Feet

Putney Mountain is both the name of a specific summit and the name of a section of north–south running ridge that becomes Windmill Ridge to the north. A small area at the summit is kept open with a combination of management and sheep grazing. The trail system crossing the mountain consists of some well-worn old hiking trails and some switchbacky newer trails as well as some sections of dirt road. The trails, which are maintained by the Putney Mountain Association (PMA), are well marked and easy to follow. This route combines the two main, generally parallel north-south trails into a moderately challenging loop that visits many of the mountain's interesting natural features. Together with a linking trail, the southernmost part of the loop forms a 1.4-mile interpretive walk called the Nature Trail. Leashed pets are permitted.

DIRECTIONS   From Putney, take Kimball Hill Road/Westminster Road north for 1.1 miles. At a fork, turn left and go 2.4 miles west on West Hill Road. Turn right and go 2.1 miles west up the hill on Putney Mountain Road. The parking area is on the right. Note that Putney Mountain Road west from the parking area is closed in winter. **GPS:** "443 Putney Mountain Road"

TRAIL   From the parking area, go north on the trail (ignoring a wide path veering off to the right) and immediately arrive at a junction with West Cliff Trail on the left. Go Straight, passing the map kiosk, and head 0.5 miles north on the white-blazed Ridgeline Trail, undulating up and down (but overall ascending) through the woods to the open

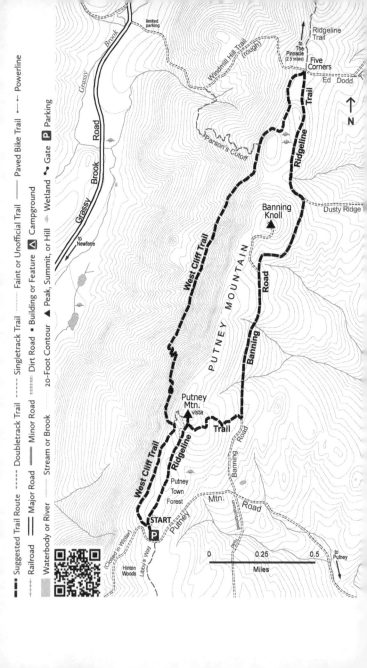

Map legend:

- Suggested Trail Route
- Railroad
- Waterbody or River
- Doubletrack Trail
- Singletrack Trail
- Stream or Brook
- Faint or Unofficial Trail
- Minor Road
- Major Road
- Dirt Road
- 20-Foot Contour
- Paved Bike Trail
- Powerline
- Building or Feature
- Campground
- Peak, Summit, or Hill
- Wetland
- Gate
- **P** Parking

N (compass, pointing up)

Grassy Brook

Grassy Brook Road

to Newfane

limited parking

Windmill Hill Trail (rough)

Parson's Cutoff

to The Pinnacle (2.5 miles)

Ridgeline Trail

Five Corners

Ed Dodd

Ridgeline Trail

Dusty Ridge

Banning Knoll ▲

West Cliff Trail

PUTNEY MOUNTAIN

Banning Road

Putney Mtn. ▲ vista

West Cliff Trail

Ridgeline

Trail

Putney Town Forest

Banning Road

START

P

Libby's Way

(Closed in Winter)

Putney Mtn. Road

to Putney

Hinton Woods

0   0.25   0.5

Miles

summit of Putney Mountain; the trail braids and rejoins itself several times in this section.

From the rock ledges at the top, backtrack a few hundred feet south into the woods, then bear left at a fork and go 0.4 miles east down the white-blazed Ridgeline Trail. After emerging from the woods and crossing under a powerline, turn left and follow Banning Road, a dirt road, north for 1.2 miles across the east side of the ridge. At a junction where the road turns right, bear left on Ridgeline Trail and go 0.6 miles north to an intersection called Five Corners at a 1,403-ft. gap. From here, the Ridgeline Trail crosses Windmill Hill Trail (an eroded old road) becomes Pinnacle Trail as it heads 2.4 miles north to the summit of The Pinnacle (see site #46).

Take a sharp left onto the yellow-blazed West Cliff Trail and run south for 2.1 miles along the sometimes steeply sloped west side of the ridge. In 0.25 miles, swing right just past a boggy wetland swale. Head due west a short distance, then curve left, traverse a hemlock-covered slope, and descend south (passing Parsons Cutoff trail on the right) at a moderate grade for about a mile along an old woods road below Banning Knoll up to the left/east. At a junction, bear left back onto narrower trail and climb up a set of switchbacks through dark hemlock forest to a junction where a steep, blue-blazed linking trail leads 0.1 mile left up to the summit of Putney Mountain.

Take a right and follow West Cliff Trail 0.6 miles south back to a junction with Ridgeline Trail. Descending slightly at first and then running mostly level, this section of the trail passes through primarily conifer woodland above cliffs and ledges, and coincides with the west half of the 1.4-mile Nature Trail interpretive loop. At the south end, go right at the junction by the kiosk to return to the trailhead.

Optional Extensions   South of Putney Mountain Road, the wide, white-blazed Libby's Way trail (formerly "Hinton Trail") leads south along the ridge for 0.7 miles on PMA land known as Hinton Woods to a T-junction where you can make various color-coded loops (blazed with small circular markers) out of the 1.5-mile Dine Trail, the beautiful 1.2-mile Hannum Trail, and the 1.6-mile Beaver Pond Loop. This trail network, which is partly on PMA land and partly on the Silvio O. Conte National Fish and Wildlife Refuge, is also accessible from southern trailheads on Holland Hill and Parkman Woods Roads (limited parking at each). All of the trails are relatively easy, though low parts may be muddy and there is some elevation change, especially along the 0.5-mile High Road Trail (which is also somewhat overgrown).

NEARBY Several miles to the east down in the valley, the **Putney Central School Forest** (owned and managed by an independent nonprofit called The Forest for Learning) features a network of color-coded loop trails on the lower western slopes of Bear Hill above Sacketts Brook (a bridge crosses the brook near the start). Parking is available at the town pool just below the school. There are also a number of other short trail systems, some on private land, scattered throughout Putney.

DISTANCE 3.4 Miles   **TOWN** Townshend

DIFFICULTY RATING Moderate   **TRAIL STYLE** Out-and-Back

TRAIL TYPE Singletrack   **TOTAL ASCENT** 1,100 Feet

Townshend State Park, originally a state forest, sits on the north-facing slope of the valley wall south of the West River. There's only one trail in the park but it's a nice one, especially good for running down once you've climbed it. The forest the trail passes through is very pretty, with several different habitat types represented, and the trail surface is generally quite easy on the feet, though there are several rooty sections and a few slippery rocks at stream crossings. While the summit of 1,680-ft. Bald Mountain is wooded now, grasses and sedges dominate the open forest floor there and scenic vistas face several different directions. Bicycles are not permitted on the trail; dogs are allowed but must be kept on a leash. Portions of this trail were badly damaged during floods in July 2023, resulting in temporary closure.

DIRECTIONS   From Rte. 30 just south of Townshend, take State Forest Road northwest for 2.7 miles (turning right at the junction with Wiswall Hill Road, which continues straight). Turn left into Townshend State Park. The parking lot is on the right.

GPS: "Townshend State Park 2755 State Forest Road"

TRAIL   The blue-blazed Bald Mountain Trail is a little tricky to find at first. The trailhead is located just to the right of the beautiful stone park office building, marked with a "Trail" sign. Descend a set of wooden steps, then turn right on the paved campground road. In a few dozen feet or so, turn left at the marked post for campsite #25. Just past the campsite entrance, the trail veers away to the right.

Descend to and cross a wooden bridge over a brook, then begin

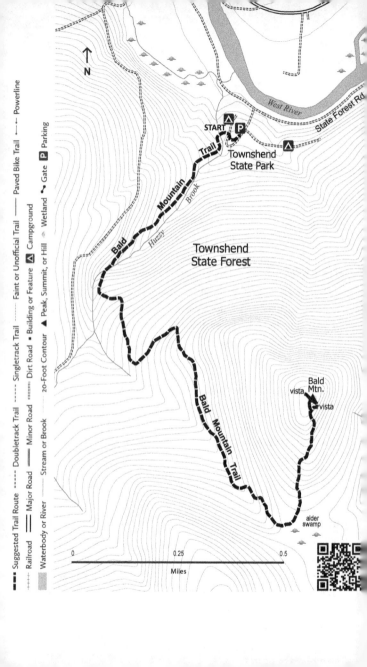

climbing uphill on the wide, soft trail hugging the slope to the right of the brook. The steep-sided stream valley is mighty scenic here, with fern-covered hillsides, mossy ledges, and pools in the stream. At around 0.5 miles, cross over the brook (may be challenging in spring or after heavy rain) and then veer left away from the brook and up the hillside, somewhat steeply at first, through northern hardwood forest.

Climb diagonally past mossy rocks across a hemlock-covered slope, then veer right at a switchback marked with an arrow at 0.75 miles and climb diagonally the other way. After a level stretch, rise southeast at a steady, gentle grade to the edge of a boggy wetland at 1.4 miles. Swing left and climb north at a steeper grade over bedrock ledges for 0.3 miles up the upper cone of the mountain to the top. Under a dry woodland canopy of oak and pine trees, the otherwise open understory here is covered in grasses and sedges, perhaps evocative of former land use when the peak was actually bald.

There are two main vistas at the summit, one to the northwest towards Stratton and Bromley near the site where a fire tower used to be, and one southeast toward Mount Monadnock. A former trail that turned this route into a loop, was closed due to severe erosion in 1996. To descend, return back the way you came, taking care to not slip on mossy rocks at the stream crossings.

NEARBY A few miles west, the 1.5-mile Ledges Overlook Hiking Trail "almost-loop" at the Army Corps of Engineers' **Townshend Lake Recreation Area** climbs somewhat steeply up a forested hillside to a scenic ledge overlooking the dam and its lake. There are two nearly adjacent trailheads near the north end of the park road.

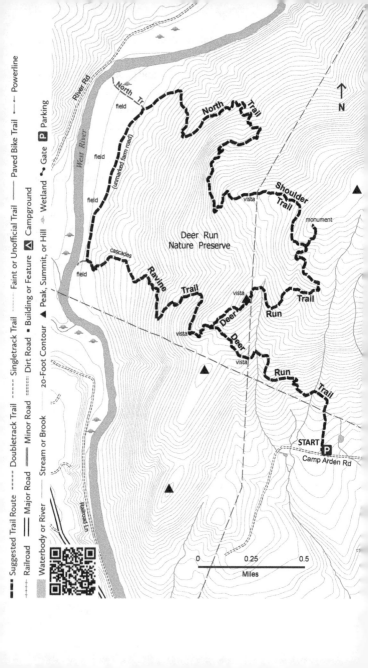

DISTANCE 6.7 Miles   **TOWN** Dummerston, Newfane, and Brookline
DIFFICULTY RATING Moderate   **TRAIL STYLE** Lollipop Loop
TRAIL TYPE Singletrack   **TOTAL ASCENT** 1,440 Feet

The relatively new Deer Run Nature Preserve hosts a very well-constructed network of marked trails that explore a steeply-sloped, rugged ridge above the West River. The trail system is maintained by the Green Mountain Conservancy (GMC), which also owns the land. The trails intentionally wander around the landscape, visiting cascades, brooks, towering trees, stone walls, riverside meadows, expansive views, and uncommon natural community habitats. This route combines many of the trails into a lollipop loop that climbs, descends, and re-climbs the ridge several times and visits a variety of interesting natural features and vistas, almost always at a gentle grade. There are multiple open powerline crossings, and a spur trail leads to a forested high point along the ridge called the "Monument" at 1,498 feet where there is a limited view through the woods. Pets are permitted but must be leashed. Bikes and horses are not allowed on these trails due to the fragility of the soils and natural habitats. More trails are planned for future development of the system.

DIRECTIONS   From Rte. 30, cross the one-lane Dummerston Covered Bridge over the West River. Immediately turn left on Camp Arden Road and go northwest for 1.9 miles (bearing left at the first fork to stay along the river) to the small but well-marked parking lot for the preserve on the right.
GPS: "Deer Run Nature Preserve, 940 Camp Arden Road, Dummerston"

TRAIL   From the trailhead, follow the blue-blazed Deer Run Trail north along the eastern edge of an open field. It starts as a narrow dirt ribbon, rising at an easy grade for 0.1 mile, subtly curving back and forth on soft ground beneath pine trees. At a junction, bear left on a wider woods road and then cross under a powerline. The trail enters the woods on the other side and narrows again.

Swing slightly left and climb northwest up the hillside at a gentle grade. At 0.25 miles, cross a bridge over a rocky seasonal stream channel. Continue climbing up the slope for 0.3 miles via a series of switchbacks and across old stone walls, then bear right at the top of a ridge of exposed bedrock and go 0.1 mile north along the ridge. Bear left down into a small valley, cross another rocky stream, then climb up to an open powerline crossing at 0.75 miles from the start. The trail through the low shrubs below the powerlines is easy to follow, but occasional trailside rocks have blue paint blazes just in case.

Reenter the woods on the west side of the powerlines and continue up the slope for about 0.25 miles to a junction with Ravine Trail on the left. Go straight to stay on Deer Run Trail and follow it northeast at a gentle grade up the ridge to another open powerline crossing. Cross a rocky knoll under the transmission lines, then descend through grassy vegetation on the other side and reenter the woods. Descend to a small stream crossing at 1.3 miles, then start up the hemlock and pine covered slope on the other side. Follow the trail uphill for 0.6 miles, swinging left around the ridge and climbing east and north to a junction.

Stay straight and follow Deer Run Trail 0.1 more miles up to its terminus at a monument on the pine-covered shoulder of the ridge where there is a limited view through the trees. It is 2 miles from the trailhead to the "Monument." From here, backtrack 0.1 mile down to the junction.

Take a right and follow the yellow-blazed Shoulder Trail 0.4 miles west to yet another open powerline swath where the trail name changes. Cross beneath the powerlines and descend the blue-blazed North Trail for 1.7 meandering miles. The somewhat rugged but easy to follow trail intentionally swings back and forth across the slope, visiting various natural features and taking its time to drop down the northwest side of the hill. At the bottom, the trail arrives at an active agricultural field south and east of the West River.

At a junction where North Trail crosses the field to the riverbank on a farm road, go left and follow a wide, grassy, and mostly flat farm road south for 0.7 miles along the east edge of the field. At a junction where a short spur leads right down to the river, take a left.

Follow the orange-blazed Ravine Trail a few hundred feet east across a field, then up into the woods. Climb at a moderate grade along the side of a steeply sloped ravine with a cascading stream babbling far down below to the left. After veering away from and leaving the ravine, the trail swings left and follows an old road gradient diagonally up the hillside, then veers right off of it and climbs to another one and does the same thing. Eventually it swings right and rises south along a conifer-covered slope to the edge of a powerline crossing. From here, the trail swings left and winds its way up through an uncommon hickory woodland with a soft, grassy understory along the crest of the ridge, then levels off and reaches a junction.

It is 1.1 miles from the West River up to the junction on the ridge. To return, take a right on Deer Run Trail for the mile-long descent back down to the trailhead.

NEARBY A few miles to the southwest across the West River and up Rock River, **Newfane Town Forest** near Williamsville features a small network of hilly, well-marked trail loops accessible from a dirt parking lot next to the town garage along Depot Road. Off Depot Road near Rte. 30, there are popular swimming holes on Rock River Preservation land where the Rock River flows through a narrow gorge. A trail that begins wide and easy becomes rocky and narrow as it visits a series of open pools (note: clothing has traditionally been optional after the first pool). Parking is by the bridge along Rte. 30.

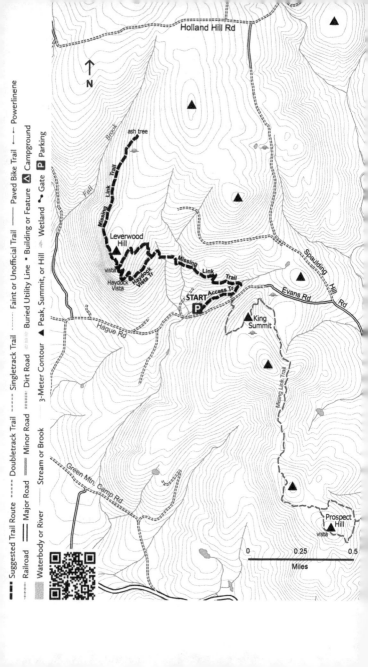

DISTANCE 3.7 Miles   **TOWN** Dummerston
DIFFICULTY RATING Moderate   **TRAIL STYLE** Out-and-Back
TRAIL TYPE Singletrack   **TOTAL ASCENT** 470 Feet

The Missing Link Trail, which is managed by Putney Mountain Association (PMA), serves as the spine of a new trail system that connects Prospect Hill in Dummerston to a point on a hillside to the north that is not far from PMA's two Holland Hill Road trailheads. PMA opened Missing Link Trail in 2020 and ultimately plans to connect it with existing networks. This suggested route follows the northern half of Missing Link Trail from a parking area along Hague Road up to the state's second largest white ash tree and the trail's temporary terminus. It passes a pair of south-facing scenic vistas on the side of Leverwood Hill, crosses a few stony brooks, and visits a number of large old trees. Bikes and dogs are permitted, and the trails are used by cross-country skiers and snowshoe hikers in the winter.

DIRECTIONS   From Rte. 30, cross the one-lane Dummerston Covered Bridge over the West River. Immediately turn left on Camp Arden Road and go northwest for 0.5 miles along the river. Bear right on Green Mountain Camp Road and go 0.2 miles up the hill. Turn left and go up Hague Road for 1.3 miles. Just before the road ends, the small parking lot is on the left (look for the hand-painted "Trail Parking" sign). Parking is a bit tight.
GPS: "645 Hague Road"

TRAIL   From the map and information kiosk at the trailhead, head 0.2 miles up the hill along a fern-lined old road grade, which is an access route to a junction. Take a left and follow the white-blazed Missing Link Trail (abbreviated as MLT on some trail signs) for 0.7

miles at a moderate grade up through northern hardwood forest to a junction.

Bear left onto the orange-blazed Haydock Vista Trail and rise gradually for 0.3 miles to 1,190-ft. Haydock Vista, a bedrock ledge in a partial clearing. From here, the wide-ranging view out across the West River valley below includes three states: Vermont, New Hampshire, and Massachusetts. The trail and vista were named for Roger Haydock, the designer, planner, and principal builder of many of the new trails in the region, including this one (though many hardworking PMA volunteers should also be credited for the work). Behind the vista, swing right and climb a set of ledges up to a junction at 1,290 feet where you'll rejoin Missing Link Trail at another, more limited vista.

Turn left and follow Missing Link Trail 0.7 miles north across and then up the hemlock-covered hillside above the Fall Brook stream valley downslope to the left. After rising gently up through a sometimes wet and seepy section, the trail dead-ends (for now) at Vermont's second-largest white ash tree, particularly impressive in its wide girth and gnarly upper branches. The trail currently ends at the tree, but it is being extended northwest up to Holland Hill Road.

To return to the Hague Road trailhead, turn around and go south on the Missing Link Trail, this time staying left at the junction with Haydock Vista Trail for a slightly shorter (0.3 miles) northern branch that descends via a series of switchbacks through a sugar maple woodland with a delightfully fern-filled understory.

Optional Extension   At the junction with the spur trail to the parking area, continue south on the Missing Link Trail; climb up a set of well-built crib steps, cross Hague Road (a woods road at this spot), and follow the trail for 0.4 miles up to the wooded top of King Summit. From there, curve right and go south for 1.5 miles to 1,167-ft. Prospect Hill. In this section, the trail crosses private lands on a mix of new singletrack and wide woods roads, rising and falling numerous times along the ridge, sometimes quite steeply. At the southern end, the

Prospect Hill Trail and Prospect Hill Trail Alternative form a hilly, 0.6-mile loop, and a 0.4-mile spur trail descends eastward to a trailhead at Park Laughton Road. A large open meadow at the top of Prospect Hill affords fine views in multiple directions, including east towards Mount Monadnock. Note that there is no parking at the southern trailhead; parking for Prospect Hill is about half a mile south near the town offices in Dummerston Center. Total out-and-back distance from Hague Road to the Prospect Hill Loop is 4.4 miles.

NEARBY In the near future, when the Missing Link Trail connects to the "Hinton Woods" network south of Putney Mountain, it will be possible to follow trails 27 miles north from Dummerston Center to the village of Grafton.

A few miles south, 1,204-ft. **Black Mountain** in Dummerston is a volcanic ring-dike looming above the West River. It features a fantastic 3–4-mile trail loop up to semi-open ledges near the top, and is accessible from two different trailheads. *Note, however, that running is prohibited on the trails of this preserve.* A relatively easy 0.6-mile trail on private land on the east side of the mountain leads to views from the sparsely wooded ledge outcrops of 1,150-ft. **Little Black Mountain**.

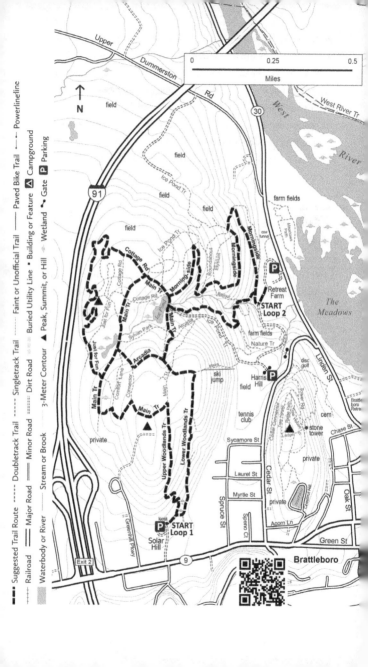

DISTANCE Loop 1: 2.2 Miles; Loop 2: 3.2 Miles   **TOWN** Brattleboro

DIFFICULTY RATING Easy/Moderate   **TRAIL STYLE** Loops

TRAIL TYPE Singletrack   **TOTAL ASCENT** Loop 1: 250 Feet; Loop 2: 360 Feet

The Retreat Trails are a connected system of paths in the hills above downtown Brattleboro. Originally created in the 1800s by the Brattleboro Retreat, the now 10-mile network has served the local community as a free public resource ever since. In recent years, volunteers rehabilitated many of the trails and new signage has been added throughout to aid with navigation. Most trails are unblazed, but there are signs at every junction, and there are a lot of junctions. There are multiple trailheads, with the three primary ones at the Retreat Farm at the north end, the Harris Hill lot in the middle, and the Solar Hill lot at the south end. In the middle of the site, the Brattleboro Outing Club's Harris Hill Ski Jump looms high above an open field; a pedestrian staircase climbs the hill alongside it. The suggested loop routes here sample a variety of the site's trails. Loop 1 combines the 1.2-mile Woodlands Interpretive Trail and the mile-long Main Trail loop and generally involves more gradual elevation changes and less climbing overall. Loop 2 is more challenging, climbing up singletrack trails from the farm and circling around the western edge of the property before descending back to the farm via a series of long, well-graded switchbacks. Along the way on each loop, many unmarked side trails lead out to private land; there is no public access on these paths so please only enter from the marked trailheads.

DIRECTIONS   LOOP 1   From I-91 Exit 2, go east on Rte. 9 for 0.2 miles. Turn left at the sign for Solar Hill and go left up the unnamed dirt road. The parking lot and trailhead are at the top.

GPS: "Retreat Farm woodland trailhead"

LOOP 2 From downtown Brattleboro, take Rte. 30/Linden Street 0.5 miles northwest to the Retreat Farm entrance on the left. Park in the designated lot on the left.

GPS: "Retreat Farm Brattleboro"

TRAIL   LOOP 1 From the Woodlands Interpretive Trail kiosk at Solar Hill, take the path northeast down into the woods. At the first junction, go right on Lower Woodlands Trail. After passing to the right of a frequently ponded swale, turn left at an unmarked junction. Climb briefly to another wet swale on the left and stay straight at an unmarked junction where a faint path leads left. Ignoring several unmarked side paths leading out to private property on the right, stay on this trail for 0.5 miles as it meanders back and forth across a gully and climbs north at a gentle grade up to a junction. On the right, a short spur leads east up to the top of the Harris Hill Ski Jump. Bear left at the junction and follow the Woodlands Trail west over to a junction with Main Trail by the end of a stone wall.

Go right and follow Main Trail north, staying on it at numerous junctions: with Arcadia on the left, then Arcadia on the right, Sylvan Park on the left, and Ice Pond on the right. The small Ice Pond will be on the left. Then pass Morningside Trail on the right and the start of Cottage Road on the left. The trail becomes somewhat grassy here. At a fork, bear left up the hill to stay on Main Trail. Bear left at another fork with Ridge Run, then stay straight at a junction with the end of Cottage Road. Soon after, curve left and cross over Cottage Road (yes, again) at an intersection, then go south to the east side of another small pond.

Stay straight on Main Trail at junctions with Arcadia on the left and Just for Fun on the right, then take a left at a junction and climb to a junction with Comfort Lane. Go right and climb to a junction with The Connector trail. Take one more right and climb up and over a wooded ridge to a junction with Upper Woodlands Trail. Take a right and follow Upper Woodlands 0.5 miles south, descending gently at first and then slightly steeper down a set of switchbacks, to a junction with Lower Woodlands Trail. Go right to return to the Solar Hill trailhead.

LOOP 2   From the Retreat Farm, follow the access road southwest past several farm buildings. At the end of the last building, just as the road begins to bear left and climb a slope to an upper field called Hope Garden, take a sharp right and follow signs pointing to Retreat Trails up the wide dirt road. Just past a subtle landscape sculpture called The Fiddlehead on the left, take a left at a junction onto the narrow Nature Trail. Blazes are small red diamond markers with white maple leaves. Follow Nature Trail across the fern-covered slope through a hemlock forest, passing a junction with Bailout Trail on the right, which leads up the hill on a wooden stairway. After weaving back and forth and up and down a bit (see figure 11), take a right on an unmarked trail (if you reach another wooden stairway at the base of a trail called Skyline Spur, you've gone too far).

Climb up the hillside on the unnamed trail at a steady, moderate grade to a junction at Ice Pond that's around 0.6 miles from the start. Go left a few feet, cross a stream, then bear right to stay on Main Trail. Stay straight at a junction with Sylvan Park on the right, then take a right on Arcadia/Main Trail and climb to a junction. Take a right on Arcadia, pass junctions with The Connector and Comfort Lane trails on the left, then descend slightly to a pond and go left/south on Main Trail (yes, Main Trail again; it's a loop and this is the other side).

After about 0.1 mile, take a right on Just For Fun, a slightly narrower and more undulating trail. At the first junction, go left onto an unnamed singletrack trail. Bear right at an unmarked junction and follow the trail north. The trail winds around a lot, climbing and descending the ridge several times. In rapid succession, stay left at two junctions with unmarked trails leading right. Follow the trail down, across, around, and up the hillside some more. At a junction, go left and follow the trail up to a junction with Cottage Road.

Take a left on Cottage Road and go southeast to a junction with Main Trail. Take a left and then an immediate right and drop down the hill to Ice Pond. Take a left onto Morningside Trail and immediately cross a wooden boardwalk bridge over a wet area. From here, follow Morningside all the way back down the hillside to the trailhead at the Retreat Farm. The descent via multiple long switchbacks is gradual, even briefly rising on occasion, with excellent soft footing the whole way, and it is very runnable and fun.

Optional Extensions

1. From the Harris Ski Jump lot in the center of the Retreat Trails system, you can make a fun short loop up on Chestnut Hill east of Cedar Street. Cross the road and climb the hill via Tower Road or Tower Climb to the stone tower near the top, then circle around the hill on Ledge Trail, Ridge Path, or Tree House Trail.

2. Another interesting extension option is to go north from the lower Retreat Farm parking area, following signs to Meadow Pathways, and take the low "cow tunnel" culvert underneath Rte. 30 to a series of loop trails around the fields between the road and the West River. Land managers are currently considering options for ultimately linking the Retreat Farm trails here directly to the east end of the West River Trail across the river. At present, the recently upgraded Hogle Trail traces the southeastern shoreline of The Meadows marsh.

3. Finally, the narrow, 0.65-mile Nature Trail traces an arc directly above the upper part of the Retreat Farm and makes a great introductory foray into running hilly, swooping singletrack trails.

NEARBY Several miles northwest, the **Hillwinds Trails** network in northern Brattleboro features several miles of easy to moderate scenic trail loops over and around a forested ridge. About a mile southwest, there is a short, somewhat confusingly marked trail network around the disc-golf course at Brattleboro's **Living Memorial Park**. Two miles south, the Sunset and Sunrise Trail loops can be combined for a short, scenic run at **Fort Dummer State Park**.

Several miles southwest, the **Sweet Pond Trail** at **Sweet Pond State Park** in Guilford makes an easy, 1.3-mile loop around a small pond. To the southeast, there are about 3 miles of short, interesting trail loops at the **Vernon Town Forest** (a.k.a. J. Maynard Miller Forest) Black Gum Swamp.

Just across the Connecticut River in New Hampshire, a trail with runnable switchbacks climbs to a vista on **Wantastiquet Mountain** in Hinsdale/Chesterfield; on the backside of the mountain, the 50-mile, long-distance **Wantastiquet-Monadnock Trail (WMT)** leads east to **Mine Ledge**, **Indian Pond**, **Madame Sherri Forest**, the **Ann Stokes Loop**, **Mount Pisgah**, and beyond.

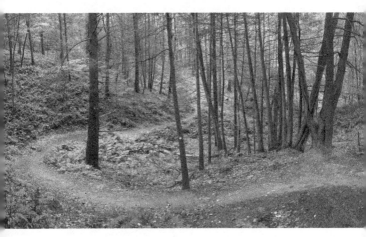

FIGURE 11. The Nature Trail at the Retreat Farm in Brattleboro.

Ben Kimball is a New England-based writer, runner, editor, and photographer. He is the author of a series of regional trail running guides and co-author of a natural history book about New Hampshire. He has written numerous articles about running and environmental issues in the northeast, and has had photos published in many local and national magazines and websites.